The Principles and Practice of

No Hands Massage

Zero-Strain Bodywork

Gerry Pyves

Shi'Zen Publications

Published by Shi'Zen Publications
The Coach House, Parkton Grove, Hangingstone Road, Berry Brow,
Huddersfield HD4 7QU

Drawings by John Coombes

Printed in Great Britain by The Charlesworth Group, Huddersfield

ISBN 0-9539074-0-6

Warning

The techniques outlined in this book are potentially injurious when used by untrained practitioners. This book in no way endorses the reader to practise these techniques, and the author accepts no liability for any damage that irresponsible practitioners may cause using them without proper training. Training in No Hands Massage® is available through Shi'Zen Ltd, the training company for No Hands Massage® - tel 01484 661600, fax 01484 667241, email office@shizen.co.uk.

Contents

PART 4
CLINICAL CONSIDERATIONS AND
THE BENEFITS OF NO HANDS MASSAGE 116

Foreword

There are few health care professions (apart from nursing perhaps) where wear and tear more rapidly manifests than in those offering therapeutic massage. Much of the damage occurs through inappropriate self-use, poor posture and inappropriate body mechanics. Much of the tissue irritation which results involves repetitive strain of key areas of the hands and arms, with the thumbs, fingers and wrists commonly exhibiting irritation, inflammation - and worse, in many therapists and practitioners. Some techniques are of course potentially more damaging than others, with deep tissue work carrying major risks to the wellbeing of the hands and arms.

Thankfully, after 40 years of regularly applying a range of soft tissue manipulation methods including, at times, deep tissue neuromuscular work, my own therapeutic instruments (ie my hands) remain functional and (relatively) undamaged. In fact they are more stressed by keyboard work, but that is another story and another book ! My relatively healthy hands and arms are, I believe, the result of a combination of good fortune (genetic characteristics) and the instillation of Alexander technique principles during my training by tutors who applied many of the principles which Gerry Pyves expounds so well in this book. I was, in effect, taught how to use my body efficiently with minimal stress. In addition I learned that by 'meeting and matching' soft tissue tensions, and varying the pressure being applied, often by assiduous use of body weight, rather than force, my digital contacts could achieve a relatively non-stressful means of addressing local dysfunction. My students will attest to the fact that I often admonish them to use their hands and body less stressfully, with the same term which was growled at me so often as a student, "Use yourself more efficiently, you'll last longer that way!" And indeed I have, and fortunately, as an osteopath, my work does not involve spending 50 or 60 minutes applying my hands to each patient's body, as do massage therapists, so reducing enormously the potential stress on my own soft tissues and joints.

Many of the principles and practices of safe self-use in the bodywork setting, which I was taught, are indeed still taught in some training programmes, most notably those involving neuromuscular therapy in the USA. (Chaitow and Delany 2000). But it is a matter of regret for most massage therapist that such education and practices do not seem to be the norm. The rate of attrition amongst bodyworkers in general, and massage therapists in particular, is extremely high, as evidenced by a recent survey (Watson 2000) which showed that over 75% of more than 250 therapists, reported bodily 'injury' as a result of their work, much of this involving the hands or arms. The problem has become so widespread that, following her own bad experience, therapist Lauriann Greene (1995) was inspired to write an excellent book for other therapists on how to go about saving their hands!

Part of the problem according to the author of this text, Gerry Pyves, lies in sheer overuse (and he explores the reasons for this), as well as a failure to use the body appropriately. His solutions are not evolutionary, they are revolutionary, since they remove the hands from much of the labour to which they are subjected in standard massage and bodywork environments.

This may appear to be a contradiction in terms, since it is reasonable to ask, 'how can you massage without using your hands ?'

Well, Gerry Pyves has used his personal experience of an overused and painful wrist, to evolve, over a period of years, a series of answers to the problems raised by the ubiquitous problem of excessive wear and tear. These answers are not only sensible, but are essentially practical and apparently not difficult to learn (and there are numerous well designed exercises in the book to help in this process). The new methods advocated do not remove the hands from the role of palpation and assessment, of course, but offer a range of alternative ways of achieving the objectives of massage, by using a surprising variety of different aspects of the arm, accompanied by skilful use of force application, involving positioning and repositioning of the therapists body.

Gerry Pyves has based much of his work on methods deriving from Oriental bodywork concepts, which have strong echoes in the systems derived by Feldenkrais and Alexander. These can usefully be summarised by the term 'the principle of least effort', which suggests that we should use the least amount of energy to achieve the maximum positive effect. The descriptions the author offers as to how to learn to use the body more efficiently during the application of treatment are very well constructed, and should be achievable by anyone who wishes to make these sensible changes.

Careful body positioning, correct angles of the application of force, together with the appropriate transfer of body weight, can in combination create an irresistible force for change in tense and tight tissues, without undue strain on the practitioner.

These are principles enshrined in good bodywork tactics, although they are not always adequately taught, and based on the evidence as to the rate of self-injury to the hands and arms, are certainly not always practised. What Gerry Pyves brings, literally, to the (treatment) table, and to the reinforcement of these good practices, is the possibility of saving the therapists hands for delicate work, by not involving them in heavy work, where safe, efficient alternatives exist.

This is a timely and well constructed book which offers a range of thoughtful and sometimes provocative choices. It is up to the reader to apply those elements which seem to best reflect opportunities for optimal self-use. Out of these energy saving approaches both the patient/client and the therapist must benefit. Hopefully teachers of massage will incorporate into their teaching many of the ideas and methods which Gerry Pyves has distilled into this book.

Leon Chaitow
Senior Lecturer, University of Westminster, London
Editor, Journal of Bodywork and Movement Therapies

Preface

The Shi'Zen of Bodywork

Calling all Bodyworkers!

This book is written to you, respected colleague, because I want to share with you a wonderful system of massage and movement that will help you to remain effective without damaging yourself.

You provide a wonderful service to your clients, as a 'purveyor of touch' in a touch-starved world. You are a valuable resource to humanity. This book acknowledges your importance, and is designed to help you protect the wonderful work that you do.

As a bodyworker, you deserve the greatest possible protection for your own body. How else can you grow old and wise and become a master of your profession?

Shi'Zen is the ancient Japanese word meaning "The elemental balance of nature". How else can this touch-starved planet find its much-needed ecological balance, its Shi'Zen, unless we bodyworkers live long and become masters of the balance that healing touch can bring to the world?

How easy would it be for the world's leaders and corporate power-mongers to make their insane decisions to wage war, despoil the planet, and ruin people's lives if they had just had a truly healing bodywork session? Their imbalances would be addressed, their needs met, their anxieties soothed. From such a Shi'Zen, truly creative decisions would emerge.

This book, then, is about prolonging and improving your health so that you can continue to provide your healing Shi'Zen to the world into your dotage. It is written for those of you who may have inadvertently damaged yourself through your bodywork. If you have ever experienced the slightest twinge, ache or pain in your body before, during or after your bodywork, then you could be in this category. This book is also for you, if you have not been injured, for here is an effective way to stay injury-free throughout the rest of your career.

Respected and valued colleagues, I offer No Hands Massage to you as one way in which you can further enhance and develop the Shi'Zen of your bodywork, to the benefit of us all.

Namaste

Gerry Pyves

Acknowledgement

I acknowledge all the clients who turned up for sessions with me and allowed me to play practitioner whilst they played client. Their bodies brought these strokes out of my body.

I acknowledge all the students who attended my monthly groups in which these ideas were tested and changed. Their faithful love and their ideas are written into every page. I would especially like to acknowledge John, Gilli, Dory, Jutika, Suzie, Anne and Geraldine for their continual challenge, their beautiful creativity, their heartfelt loyalty, and for their belief in me.

I acknowledge all the wonderful teachers who have had such a personal direct influence on my bodywork, my communications and my thinking. Especially I thank Ron Rieck, Sonia Moriceau, Don McFarland and Dave Spenceley. I also acknowledge all the great innovators and pioneers of bodywork throughout history who were influencing my bodywork even when I did not know it.

I acknowledge all the people who have helped make this book a reality. Diane Watson for her gentle power and making it all happen. Stephanie Smith for her sense of humour whilst putting it all together, and the whole Shi'Zen team for their love and support.

Dedication

I dedicate this book to my wife Francesca who has supported me and loved me, even when times were hard. You listened when no one was listening.   You believed in me and loved me even when I did not believe in or love myself. I also dedicate this book to my children Laurie, Hannah and Alfie. You teach me the important things in life – how to love and keep on loving and never to lose the faith.

Introduction

Out of the Ashes. . .

It was a cold and wet November morning and I awoke with a deep aching pain in my right wrist. My first thought was "How can I massage eight clients today?". During breakfast I tested the extent of damage to my wrist by lifting my mug of tea. . . "Ouch!". A shooting pain up my arm made me grimace. This was not a good sign. It was Friday morning, and I had completed three out of four days of my weekly massage clinic .

I looked across the table at my son, Laurie, two years old, covering his face with raspberry yoghurt without a care in the world. I looked at my partner Francesca, talking about her day, enjoying this precious time when we were all together. I looked around at our small London flat, and began to worry about paying the mortgage.

After six years of building a massage practice I was now seeing 25 - 30 clients a week, yet I was still struggling to bring home much money after the costs of renting, advertising and maintaining a treatment room in West Hampstead, London. Francesca was doing some part-time work and we were already feeling the pressure of this. The thought of cancelling clients scared me as I calculated that my earnings so far this month would not even cover my overheads. I also knew that the deep aching pain I was experiencing was a result of cumulative strain on the tendons and ligaments of my wrist, and this could mean enforced rest. So I sat there in the kitchen and silently panicked.

This wrist problem was not new. Over the previous year I had increasingly experienced the warning signs of stiffness and aching in my thumbs and wrists. My clients demanded my very best, and that's what I gave them. It just seemed impossible to do effective bodywork without causing myself pain - despite all my hand stretching and strengthening exercises, my focus on 'good posture', and my use of all the smart body-saving techniques I had come across.

This morning was different. Today I had entered the realms of sharp debilitating pain. As I travelled the tube from Brixton to West Hampstead, I wanted to hold and support my wrist in a protective sling. I felt vulnerable to knocks and bumps. As I checked messages on my clinic ansafone, I found myself wishing for eight cancellations. No such luck! As my first client sat down and started talking about himself I found myself wondering if I could suggest some relaxation exercises and de-stressing visualisations instead of bodywork.

With a growing sense of despair I heard Anton, a 16 stone concert musician, requesting deep structural massage and I found myself automatically going through the routine of leaving him to get undressed and on to the couch. I knew I should be cancelling and yet I balked at giving up without a fight. I did not want to lose the business and income that my family and I had spent the last six years building up.

I entered the room and placed my hands gently on Anton's back. . . maybe I could do some gentle healing work..., let that warm magic of touch do the work today. . . No way. His body was screaming "TENSION!!!!". If Anton's body had got up off the table and demonstrated his needs that day, he would have been on his hands and knees begging me to apply that deep releasing pressure that only massage can provide.

So I started working and kneading his armour-plated spinal muscles with my left hand, providing what I was persuading myself was "psychological reassurance" by resting my injured right hand gently on his back. "Anyway", I convinced myself, "I work too much with my right hand, it would be good to focus on 'leading with my left', and strengthen up my left side to achieve greater balance. . ."

Within a few minutes I realised that I was just not providing Anton with the massage he deserved. Was it my imagination or was there a questioning silence in his body, as if to say "Why are you only working with one hand?". I also started to feel pain in my left wrist. "Great! What am I supposed to do now?"

I finally faced reality, decided to concede defeat and apologise to Anton and cancel the session. . . and the rest of my clients for the day. . . and probably the rest of the month. . . My mind started to wander over any loan options I could think of to cover my costs this month, wishing I'd had the money to take out that insurance policy to cover me for the time off through sickness or injury.

In despair I leaned my forearms on his back and took a deep breath of resignation. Panicky visions of repossession and bankruptcy flooded my mind. As I exhaled, I felt like crying and slumped a little more on to my forearms, all thoughts of massage gone from my mind. I had entered my dark hole of despair from which the panic had sought to protect me. Lou Reed's "This is the end, my friend" would have been a fitting accompaniment to my mood at this moment. I was sinking into a darkness, far away from the massage room. . .

From somewhere in the distance I heard Anton saying "Ooooh, that's just great. . . mmmm". As if coming out of a dream, I took in what Anton had said. Coming to, and opening my eyes, I realised I had practically collapsed my whole body-weight on to my forearms, leaning on his back. Confused, I leaned a little harder and he made more satisfied noises. I started to lean on and off his body and he kept going "Yes! Wow! Brilliant!". Excitement started to replace despair inside me. I suddenly remembered my first massage tutor once showing me how to use my forearm down the back, and copied this - the only No Hands stroke I knew. I rubbed oil into my forearms and started to explore the different surfaces that were available to me by using this part of my body. I began to notice how differently I moved my body in order to produce massage strokes, and I began to think about other areas of my body I could use to apply pressure to Anton's screaming back. Only it wasn't screaming anymore. Anton's back was purring with delight. I had begun to dance the dance of No Hands Massage.

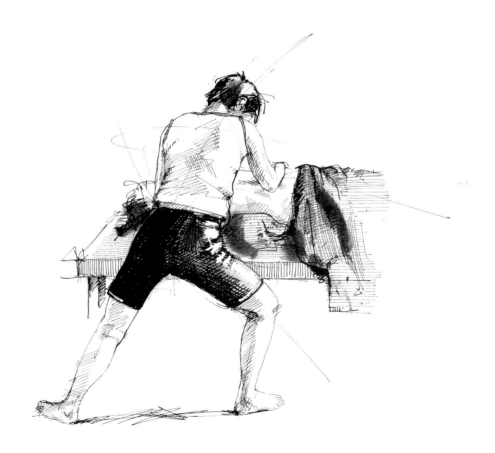

Eight years and over 5000 No Hands Massages later I sit, at 5.00 am, writing this in my attic in the tiny town of Hebden Bridge in the South Yorkshire Pennines. My wrists have never hurt since that day (except once after playing football, and more recently when holding up both my older children to watch the millennium fireworks celebrations on the Thames in London for 20 minutes!). More than that, I have found that the act of using my whole body differently has actually had a beneficial and healing effect on my body. Massaging with the rest of my body has meant that I have been constantly engaged in a creative way with my client's body and my own. The increased use of the forearm means that the very muscles which had been tight *in my own arm* are now being massaged by my clients as I massage them.

Now, my massage has transformed itself into a daily self-healing exercise for me as well as for my clients. I move and breathe differently, I enjoy my own body's movements whilst massaging, and I work effortlessly. I look forward to each bodywork session with a combination of selfish and altruistic pleasure. My clients often feel "complete" and "well worked" with much shorter sessions, and I can now go on for much longer! After each session I feel as if I have attended a Tai Chi movement and meditation session, a Yoga class and a work out in the Gym all rolled into one. I am healthier, fitter and more flexible than at any time before in my life. The massage graduates I mentor have all reported similar results from their own experiences.

If you are a bodyworker who has ever felt the slightest twinge, ache or pain in your body, then this book is written for you.

Gerry Pyves, Hebden Bridge 2000

自然

PART 1   THE PRACTITIONER'S BODY

Chapter 1   From Technique to Therapy

The Historical Perspective(1)

Per Henrik Ling (1776 - 1839) is generally considered to be the 'father' of modern western massage. His system of exercise and movement therapy incorporated massage techniques which became the basis of most later writings on massage. This was known as the Swedish movement cure, and is what we now call 'Swedish Massage'.

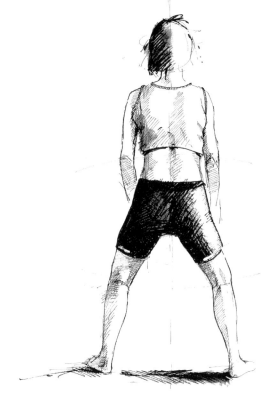

Dr Mathias Roth, an English physician who studied directly with Ling brought this cure to England just after Ling's death and published the first book on the subject in 1850. Others took the cure to Russia, Germany and Austria. This western system of massage was introduced into America in 1856 by two brothers, Charles F Taylor and George H Taylor, who had learned their skills from Dr Roth in England. Van der Why (1994).

The more medical strand of massage history can be traced through Dr Johann Mezger of Holland (1829 - 1909). He brought massage techniques to the attention of the scientific community as a form of medical treatment. It is his followers who used the French terms *effleurage*, *petrissage* and *tappotment friction* and *vibration*, to describe massage techniques. The reason for this is unclear, but was in keeping with the practice of the international scientific community of the nineteenth century in using French as their primary international language.

The five foundation techniques of *effleurage, petrissage, tappotment, vibration* and *friction,* then, have evolved from this historical background. These are the core techniques still taught to this day in most massage schools.

What can be seen and read in the writings of Mezger *and in the majority of subsequent literature* is an almost exclusive emphasis on the use of the hands and fingers for the application of massage techniques. Famous massage authors such as Max Bohm, Mary McMillan, Edgar Cyriax and many others have followed on with this assumption - that the hands are the primary part of the body to be used for the application of massage techniques(2). Any visit to a modern day bookstore and a quick browse through the massage books on sale will provide the reader with ample evidence of the continuity of this tradition.

The majority of advanced massage and soft-tissue techniques that have evolved during the last century, many of which involve deep tissue work, also emphasise the hands for their technical application(3). Many of the innovative developments in bodywork, such as Rolfing, for example, have likewise continued in this tradition, at a time when better alternatives for the practitioner existed(4).

Whilst some creative massage authors with clear clinical experience have included photographs or pictures of the use of the forearms for massage, there has not been a very thorough analysis of the techniques involved. Nor am I aware of any published questioning of this professional '*Credo* of the hand' which is still being taught daily in most massage and bodywork schools throughout the world.

Recently, articles and books have begun to appear highlighting the increasing number of injury problems that conventional massage techniques are producing in practitioners. In the light of this, and on the basis of my own and my clients' positive experiences of using different techniques, I think it is an appropriate time to ask the following question:

>*"On what grounds do we continue to emphasise the almost exclusive use of the hands for the application of massage techniques?"*

Why No Hands?

Most of the arguments used to justify the continuing use of outdated techniques, first systematised almost 200 years ago by Ling, are based on the profession's need for dexterity and sensitivity. Whilst it is true that the hand is clearly the most dexterous part of the body, and provides the best surface for subtle palpation, this does not justify the *exclusivity* of the hand in conventional massage approaches. There are many creative ways in which the practitioner can ethically and professionally use other parts of the body to apply massage strokes.

Moreover, the majority of massage techniques require neither complex dexterity nor purely palmar sensitivity. As will be seen in the section on the postural principles, I am a passionate protector of the sensitive hand. Under current conditions, this is the part of the body which the profession is actually injuring!

My intention is to help preserve the hands and backs of as many practitioners of this creative profession as possible. The use of other parts of the body ensures that the hands are protected precisely so that they can be used for what they are best at - dexterity and sensitivity.

Another problem is that the profession is still defining itself along historical medical and structural models and mainly looking to non-masseurs to lead it in its technical development and evolution. However, these structurally effective techniques are, in fact, the most demanding in terms of combining a need for sensitivity, dexterity *and pressure*, and are all designed around the client's stated outcome of wanting to fix a structural problem. The number of books on the structural and medical aspects of massage massively outnumber books on the energetic, emotional, mental and spiritual effects of massage. This medicalisation of massage, however, does not necessarily reflect the public's interest.

The experience of many massage practitioners is that clients are looking for all sorts of different desired outcomes, including nurturance, body-mind connection and detoxification - to name but a few. Because of this, massage practitioners are developing and innovating all the time in order to meet the specific needs of their modern day clients. (I deal with this more fully in the second book of this trilogy: '*Six Styles Massage*'.)

Structural, sports and medical massage, then, only represent one important aspect of massage. Yet even these structural techniques can be replaced with other techniques which do not risk damage to the hands if practitioners are willing to use their bodies differently. In fact, sports massage therapists have been the ones to embrace this new approach most readily, as it has enabled them to be more effective in their demanding and highly pressurised field of work.

The argument that the hand is gentle and conveys a reassuring human contact is missing the point. Soft and gentle touch does not need to be replaced, as this gives no stress to the practitioner's joints. When reassurance and nurturance are required then, by definition, there is no harm to the practitioner's palmar surface, fingers or wrists, and therefore there is no need for abandoning use of the hands. It is also true that many other surfaces of the practitioner's body can provide the required reassurance when applied gently and with awareness.

After more than ten years of teaching the No Hands approach, I have yet to find a conventional massage technique, manipulation or stretch that cannot be replaced by the creative and sensitive use of other parts of the practitioner's body.

Students find that by replacing conventional massage techniques with the creative application of forearm techniques and techniques using other parts of the practitioner's body, *many conventional techniques are actually improved upon*. This statement is based on the comments of practitioners and clients who have received comparative massage techniques. In addition, students report a surge of excitement and renewed interest in their work due to the 'whole body creativity' which is required when the hands are abandoned. The Seven Postural Principles outlined in this book stimulate the naturally creative instincts which most massage therapists have for devising innovative movement and treatment protocols.

A Changing Profession

One reason why the profession has stayed so loyal to the hand may now be an historical anachronism. I believe that despite a touching loyalty to traditional techniques, most massage practitioners are in fact practising *an entirely different therapy* to that outlined by the early writers.

In Per Ling's Swedish system, massage applications were only a small part of the work of the therapist. Per Ling was a person passionately interested in health, for which, interestingly, massage was only a part of his overall approach. He was in fact more interested in the prevention of illness through a combination of massage, healthy exercise and assisted movements. His work was much more akin to a modern personal sports coach or a physiotherapist, observing gymnasts going through their movements, identifying weaknesses, strengthening and stretching different muscle groups, and so on.

The more that massage has been associated with alternative medicine and holistic treatments, rather than with mainstream allopathic medicine, the more we find independent and often isolated practitioners plying their trade in private rooms and clinics. The very popular massage therapy offered by these dedicated therapists is much more geared to the needs of modern clients, for reducing psychological and emotional stress and tension, than to traditional concepts of medical cure.

Like the ancient Greeks, with their philosophy of balance, modern day massage practitioners are far more interested in the overall lifestyle habits of their clients, than in the treatment of symptomatic ailments. The increasing interest in concepts of 'holism' in most massage training establishments reflects this healthy trend.

It seems that in this modern age of massive social and technological upheaval, many empathic therapists have instinctively moved their massage away from its medical and sports roots and transformed it into a highly relevant new therapy(5). I believe that the massage profession's response to the changing needs of modern clients is partly due to the empathy of its practitioners, and partly due to the profession's historical lack of regulation(6).

As society changes, so too must its therapies. This is what massage therapists and bodyworkers have achieved over the last century.

I believe that the independent-minded nature of most of its practitioners has resulted in a profession which has been silently and humbly reinventing itself to respond to the needs of modern day men and women. I believe that this is one of the reasons why massage was recently found to be the third most popular alternative or complementary therapy in America, and why similar statistics in the UK show that more than 80% of Alternative and Complementary practitioners employ touch as their primary tool of therapy. Just under

47% of Alternative and Complementary practitioners are massage therapists, aromatherapists and reflexologists. Report to the National Institutes on Health on Alternative Medical Systems and Practices in the US (1994), Exeter's Centre for Complementary Health Studies Report (2000)

This phenomenal professional success, however, means that such practitioners may now be using their hands for up to 50 - 90 minutes per treatment. This is a very different use of massage techniques than was practised in Per Ling's day. It is also very different from massage used in allopathic settings. In these modern day medical settings, physiotherapists, osteopaths and chiropractors may be using conventional massage techniques for only a few minutes of each session.

My main contention, then, is that this is a very different use of massage techniques than was common practice in the 1820's when Per Henrik Ling was teaching his Swedish movement cure. For this reason, I believe that the very title 'Massage Practitioner' may now be an anachronism. This can be seen in the many ways in which practitioners have been reinventing themselves with new and colourful titles. This is one of the reasons for the popularity of the term 'bodyworker' which is an umbrella term covering the variety of work going on. This diversity and creativity makes our profession (whatever we call it) one of the most exciting and innovative communities to which I have ever had the privilege to belong.

The rapidly evolving and highly creative aspect of massage therapy means that it is appropriate to take a new look at traditional assumptions regarding techniques. A new way of working needs to be found for practitioners who may be using their hands exclusively for most of the session, every session of the day, most days of the week. Nor is it only the hand which becomes injured in such an intensification of the profession's use of conventional massage techniques. The awkward and unique problems posed by working around a treatment couch for most of the day is damaging practitioners' necks, shoulders, backs and hips. The result is a profession which is damaging itself.

In the next chapter I go on to explore the type of damage that practitioners are in danger of causing themselves nowadays through the use of conventional historical massage techniques.

Chapter 2   Squaring the Circle - The Postural Problems of Bodywork

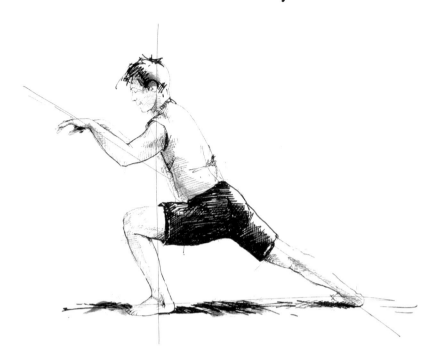

Body Posture and Hand Strain

The bio-mechanics of Bodywork present some unique and well documented postural problems due to working around a massage table. These problems tend to be focused on the back, the shoulders, the elbows and the hands. Upper body strain *can* be reduced if the best principles of movement currently available in bodywork literature are followed(1).

Such principles mainly involve protecting the practitioner's back from strain by using body-weight, rather than musculature, to transfer pressure on to the client's body. These principles also involve practitioners focusing their awareness on their own movements(2).

In this chapter I will demonstrate that use of most of the postural principles and massage techniques which trainers and writers advocate in order to protect the practitioner's back, actually results in an increase in the pressure applied to their hands, thumbs, fingers and wrists. Unfortunately, the better the practitioner's use of body-weight, the more strain is transmitted to the hands. The result is the increased risk of over-use injuries.

Cassar (1999, p.14) states that "The therapist's body-weight is used to apply pressure to the massage movement". Tappan (1988, p.13) states that "A good operator can apply pressure by a shift of body-weight instead of using muscle strength". Holey & Cook (1997, p.120) show an excellent photograph of the impossibility of good practice for conventional effleurage of the back. This photograph demonstrates the potential damage to the practitioner's back when weight is not fully transferred to the hands. Because of the unsupported lean and twist in this photograph, repetition is bound to cause strain and eventual injury. Cash (1996, p.26) states that "The good therapist. . . uses his whole body, and the hands are just the sensitive 'machine heads' that come into contact with the patient."

Beck (1988, p.334) also states that "While the hands are the main implements delivering manipulations to the client, the positioning and strength of the entire body are essential to deliver effective massages over an extended period of time.". Regarding the danger of overstrain, Holey & Cook (1997, p.162), senior physiotherapists from Norfolk UK, state that "Excessive compressive forces can cause joint injury. The wrist and joints of the fingers and thumbs are those at greatest risk when massaging.".

As long as bodyworkers are committed to using their hands, the option is either to damage the back by over-straining upper body muscles, or to damage the hands by transmitting body-weight into the hands. Either way the practitioner's body is at risk of injury. That is why I describe these principles as heroic attempts to 'square the circle' - that is, to attempt the impossible.

About Palms, Fingers, Thumbs and Wrists

Palms, fingers, thumbs and wrists are the conventional tools of bodywork. Most bodyworkers are trained to use these parts of their anatomy to achieve the results their clients desire. An analysis of any bodywork book, including shiatsu and acupressure, will show a predominance of hand and finger techniques. If I were to hazard a guess, I would place hand techniques as the primary focus of over 90% of massage and bodywork literature.

Only rarely does available literature embrace forearm strokes, and often these are photographs or drawings showing clenched fists, or use of the bony or upper part of the forearm to apply deep pressure which causes pain to the client. Where forearms are shown they are generally being used for trigger point work or friction work and, here, only the elbow *point* is favoured. For myself, this sort of deep tissue friction is precisely the sort of risky occasion where I would rather have the sensitivity of my thumb or finger available for instant bio-feedback and client protection.

Whenever bodywork involves light pressure or sensitive palpation there is no strain. However, if our bodywork requires us to transmit force through the joints and muscles of the palms, fingers, thumbs and wrists, we have a perpetual problem - a problem that has beset all bodyworkers. These joints and muscles are only small and are better suited to precise and specific work. They are also relatively fragile, and are extremely vulnerable to over-strain injuries. If they were big muscled or large boned joints they would be useless as tools of precision. How then, as bodyworkers, do we transmit force through these vulnerable parts of our bodies for six to eight hours a day, five days a week without injuring ourselves? Most writers agree that a successful practitioner will need to work for this length of time(3). However, it is important to remember that many people go into bodywork as a hobby or as part of a life-style change that does not consist of full time practice. Nonetheless, the same principles apply whether we do one or a thousand strokes a day.

This problem has exercised the creativity of bodywork trainers, practitioners and writers throughout time. How can we *transmit force* through our hands without injuring ourselves? Without the hands, how can we do bodywork? Here is my summary of the four most creative *partial* solutions to what is, I believe, an unsolvable problem.

Partial Solutions

1   Straight digits, straight arms

If we want to use fingers or thumbs *to transmit force* to the muscles and fascia of our clients, then conventional bodywork wisdom teaches us to adopt a 'straight arm posture' wherever possible. If the joints that are applying the force are in alignment with each other, and are stabilised in whatever manner possible, then sideways strain is eliminated.

This does minimise the damage that can arise if we bend our finger or thumb joints whilst applying pressure. It also aims to reduce the muscle strain and instability of flexed elbows. This approach is described and demonstrated in many manuals of massage(4).

The approach is mostly followed when we do deep work with thumbs or fingers, aligning a straight thumb with straight arm and a whole body lean.

I do agree that this is a partially protective measure. However, one simple fact is inescapable: that we are transmitting *the whole force of the stroke* (which could include our body-weight) through the tiny finger and thumb joints (inter-phalangeal joints and thenar joint).

Apart from the tension needed in the rest of the arm and upper torso muscles in holding such a stiff, unflowing posture, these joints are not designed to carry such large compressive forces. In addition, it should be said that clinically, in the often time-stressed environment of bodywork, such careful protection of thumbs and fingers is not possible.

2   Bent elbows, bent wrists

When doing lighter kneading work with fingers and thumbs, the elbows and wrists are often slightly bent. The practitioner's body is relaxed and loose in order to allow the easy transfer of weight into the fingers, thumbs and wrists. This is combined with the muscular action of the digits and thumb to produce effective bodywork. The relaxed posture of the practitioner combined with the steady and repetitive working of the client's muscle tissues with the small digital muscles is intended to reduce excessive strain. Some bodywork manuals even go into the importance for practitioners to breathe and centre themselves in order to avoid over effort and over strain(5).

Whenever we take such a relaxed and centred stance, with bent elbows and wrists, however, we trade the uncomfortable rigidity of straight arms for *extreme sideways stress* on our wrist and thumb joints due to the angle of force being applied. Not only is body-weight pressure applied into the joint every time we lean even slightly into the bodywork, but also the actions of the thumb and finger muscles in applying the massage techniques transfers this strain into horizontal movements.

In my opinion this actually doubles the strain and stress on the joint(6).

3   Bent wrists, straight arms

Another technique for effective massage, is to use the whole palm or the base of the wrist (thenar and hypo thenar eminences) to give strong and deep strokes to the client's muscles(7). This is a great technique as the whole of the practitioner's weight can be transferred into the soft tissues of the client.

This stroke enables practitioners to achieve the structural effects that clients most often desire. It is a wonderfully powerful stroke that can provide deep passive stretching and detoxification of the client's muscle fibres. It also enables the practitioner to lean into the stroke and develop a kinaesthetic 'feel' for the work through whole body movement, as well as through the hands. This body awareness, in my opinion, helps to build and develop sensitivity, intuition and - ultimately - confidence.

However, this approach creates *extreme stress on the wrist joint* produced by the combination of joint flexion and considerable body-weight. The vectors of stress to the joints are a postural nightmare which will inevitably produce strain and injury if repeated over and over again(8).

4   Knuckles

This technique, shown in some detail by Cassar (1999) attempts to solve the problem of stress to the small joints, by transferring the practitioner's body-weight on to the back of the hand.

Again, this technique is only another partial solution. It does not save the wrist joint from the considerable pressures exerted through it. In addition, in order to roll the wrists over sufficiently to perform this technique, the shoulders can easily become raised and the body posture altered, creating additional strain in the back and neck.

We still have not solved the problem of transferring force and body-weight through some of the smallest joints in the body(9).

Old Friends

As I write about each of the aforegoing strokes, I feel as if I am writing about old friends. I have felt elation at the releases I observed in my clients when I used these wonderful techniques. For years these strokes were like reliable friends. Day in and day out, they did the business. Every time I used them I felt connected with my teacher and my fellow students. I remembered what these strokes felt like on my body. I was attached to them. The bodywork techniques we use are an important and significant part of a bodyworker's life, as are the tools a mechanic uses. Like a mechanic, I would become very defensive if someone tried to take my tools away. After all, these postural solutions were what I had earned my living with! I knew they worked.

Until the morning I woke up and couldn't lift my coffee mug.

And I have since met so many bodyworkers who share a similar story.

The sadness I now feel as I point out the inadequacies of these strokes is enormous. I feel as if I am betraying old friends. For many years I was a passionate advocate and teacher of these techniques. I taught students to breathe and lean into their strokes, so they could be powerful and effective and build successful practices. Sometimes it is hard to let go of old habits, in the same way that it is hard to lose friends and move on. In my psychotherapy practice I often warn clients that if they really want to make the changes they ask for, they will probably end up changing job, changing partners, moving house and losing many friends. All change involves letting go. To cease hurting myself, I had to let go of learned techniques. I still miss them and everything I associated with them. I miss them until I think of the damage they have done to me, and of the stress they create in the wrists and hands of every bodyworker in the land who uses them.

Downward Pressure

Throughout the literature on bodywork we find many references to practitioners transferring or leaning their body-weight "into the stroke". Yet this very same pressure can only be transmitted "into the stroke" through the wrist, finger and thumb joints. No matter how well we do this work, we cannot escape the inherent strain that bodyworkers are required to place on their own joints. *It is this very transference of weight and force that powers our strokes.*

Without our body-weight we are like a stalled motorboat on a lake - idle and ineffective. Despite repeated admonitions in the better books to "only apply force in the direction of the stroke", the techniques taught actually require a *downward* pressure on to the client's body that instantly creates stress for the practitioner's wrist joint. Without this joint strain, there can be no deep bodywork.

Fritz (1995 p.184) in her 'bodymechanics...' principle no.3 states "It is important to stay behind the stroke". This 'lean in the direction of the stroke' theory seems to discount the fact that the weight of the arm and gravity do not produce enough *downward* force on the muscles to do anything more than simplyglide ineffectively across the top of the body. The direction of the stroke is not lateral, it islateral **and** downwards.

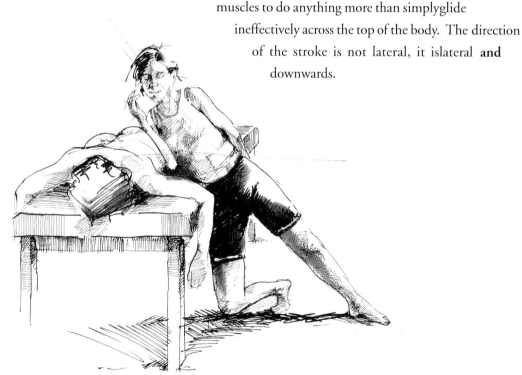

Body-weight and muscle contraction has to be applied in a downward force in order to create the stroke. The more downward pressure, the more effective the stroke. Many photographs and diagrams used to demonstrate this "behind the stroke" theory sadly fail to demonstrate the downward force required to produce an effective stroke.

Eyerman (1987, p.54-57), on the other hand, demonstrates the need for downward force for effective massage. Through stunningly beautiful photographs of his whole body movements, he provides a much truer visual impression of the amount of weight being transferred into the fingers, wrists and thumbs for powerful and effective bodywork

Zero-Strain

As I have said, in each of the above cases, the solution is only partial. What I am proposing is a *total solution* to this postural problem of bodywork - a zero-strain solution.

It makes no logical sense to apply repeated pressure on to the tiny joints of the palms, fingers, thumbs and wrists. The result for my own body after three years of full time practice was the disabling wrist pain I described in the opening of this book. It was possible to do the 'bent wrist straight arm posture' and 'knuckling'- for a while. The wrist joint is a bigger joint than the finger joints and can take greater strain, but it too will give way after the hours and months of intensive repetitive use that comes with a successful full time practice.

A total solution, then, means *totally abandoning the use of our hands* for any bodywork which requires force or pressure. Only then do we create a bodywork system that produces zero-strain for the practitioner's body.

Chapter 3　　Bodywork and Injury

Bodywork and Over-Use Injury

The use of the techniques outlined in the previous chapter, results in large forces being applied to the smallest joints, muscles, nerves and tendons of the human body (hand and fingers). This is achieved by applying body-weight and force at the same time as making massage movements with the digits or thumbs. This combination of complex and sometimes very precise digital or flexed wrist activity with abnormal weight bearing pressure is the key problem for bodyworkers. When such high-strain, high stress movements are repeated over and over, we have all the necessary pre-conditions for Over-Use Injury. Greene (1995), Adams (2000).

The trouble with Over-Use Injury is that we are dealing with repeated and on-going micro traumas to the tissues of the body. These only reveal themselves as the degenerative deformities of osteo and rheumatoid arthritis, tendonitis, repetitive strain injury, carpal tunnel syndrome and a host of other chronic conditions *many years later on*. This shocking process is outlined in the flowchart on the following page, which presents a summary of current medical understanding regarding the causes of overuse injuries.

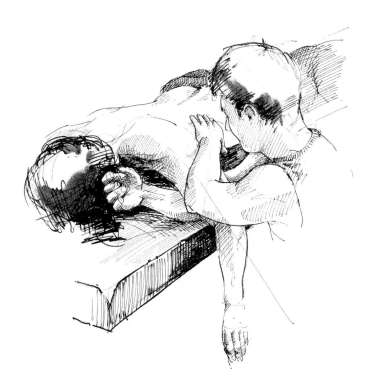

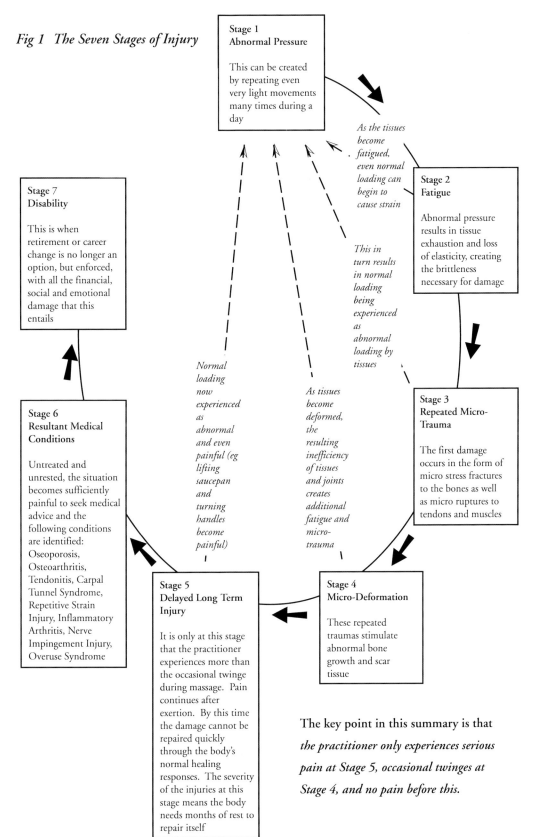

Fig 1   The Seven Stages of Injury

Stage 1
Abnormal Pressure

This can be created by repeating even very light movements many times during a day

As the tissues become fatigued, even normal loading can begin to cause strain

Stage 2
Fatigue

Abnormal pressure results in tissue exhaustion and loss of elasticity, creating the brittleness necessary for damage

This in turn results in normal loading being experienced as abnormal loading by tissues

Stage 3
Repeated Micro-Trauma

The first damage occurs in the form of micro stress fractures to the bones as well as micro ruptures to tendons and muscles

Normal loading now experienced as abnormal and even painful (eg lifting saucepan and turning handles become painful)

As tissues become deformed, the resulting inefficiency of tissues and joints creates additional fatigue and micro-trauma

Stage 7
Disability

This is when retirement or career change is no longer an option, but enforced, with all the financial, social and emotional damage that this entails

Stage 6
Resultant Medical Conditions

Untreated and unrested, the situation becomes sufficiently painful to seek medical advice and the following conditions are identified: Oseoporosis, Osteoarthritis, Tendonitis, Carpal Tunnel Syndrome, Repetitive Strain Injury, Inflammatory Arthritis, Nerve Impingement Injury, Overuse Syndrome

Stage 5
Delayed Long Term Injury

It is only at this stage that the practitioner experiences more than the occasional twinge during massage. Pain continues after exertion. By this time the damage cannot be repaired quickly through the body's normal healing responses. The severity of the injuries at this stage means the body needs months of rest to repair itself

Stage 4
Micro-Deformation

These repeated traumas stimulate abnormal bone growth and scar tissue

The key point in this summary is that *the practitioner only experiences serious pain at Stage 5, occasional twinges at Stage 4, and no pain before this.*

Even the relatively light pressure of word processing produces a high rate of occupational injury in the form of Over-Use Injury and RSI, or Repetitive Strain Injury (because word processing requires repetitive, complex movements involving manual dexterity over long periods of time). Bodyworkers are using the same dexterity, but at the same time are often applying great force in order to lengthen and soften tight and hardened muscles. This actually puts us in a much higher risk category.

To convey the seriousness of what we are doing to ourselves, I have created a formula which I call 'The Damage Formula', or 'D-Formula' for short.

The 'D-Formula'

This formula summarises the extreme danger in which practitioners place themselves whenever they apply force or pressure through their fingers, thumbs or wrists. This formula can be expressed in words as follows:

Delayed practitioner strain or damage is most likely to occur when specific hand movements are applied with abnormal force repeatedly over time.

This means that when dexterous and digital movements are repeated over and over again during each session, many sessions a day, many days a week, we generate permanent damage. This damage may only become manifest after the injury has occurred. Because of the invisibility of this micro trauma, practitioners are unaware of the damage they are doing to themselves *and continue using the same techniques*, thereby compounding the problem. In formulaic terms, when,

D = Delayed Damage (to the practitioner)
H = Hand Movements (dexterous, ie complex and specific)
AF = Applied Force (body-weight and muscles)
T = Time (repetitive: per hour, per day, per year)

then we have the following equation:

$$D = H \times AF \times T$$

In the light of this equation, unless there is a radical re-evaluation of all conventional bodywork techniques, the Massage and Bodywork profession is in danger of bequeathing an injurious legacy to all its current and future members.

Interestingly, this formula can be easily memorised by it's phonetic reading as the "Daft" formula, which is appropriate as it makes no sense for bodyworkers to cause themselves permanent injury.

Adjusting the 'D-Formula'

To transform the profession into a healthy one we need to reduce the strain. A reduction in any of the three components of this formula will produce a partial reduction in strain and therefore reduce the possibility of later injury. For example, where the applied force (AF) is light, or when our hands (H) are making simpler 'low-strain' movements, or when techniques are not repeated very often (T), then there will always be a reduction in strain.

This makes the 'D-Formula' a practical one, as practitioners can constantly remind themselves either to reduce their use of the hand, or to reduce the amount of force or to reduce the number of times certain movements are used. However, in the light of this formula, each component can be seen to only *partially* reduce the amount of damage to practitioners.

Zero-Strain – The 'Z-Formula'

If we wish to 'walk the talk' of healing and health, and eradicate all damage to ourselves as practitioners, we must change the 'D-Formula' to create zero-strain. This is achieved by eliminating the use of our hands completely, for all techniques requiring pressure. Thus,

> *To completely eradicate the possibility of any future injury to the hands and wrists, we simply replace the use of our Hands ('H') with other, stronger and less vulnerable parts of our body, ie 'No Hands' ('NH'). This creates a new formula, which we may call the 'Zero-Strain Formula' or the 'Z-Formula'.*

We do this by introducing other surfaces of the body which can achieve the desired therapeutic results equally well. When an equation uses a "0" multiplication on one side of the equation, it produces a result equalling Zero. This is because Zero multiplied by Zero equals Zero.

So too, by withdrawing the hands completely from the equation, we create a formula:

$$Z \text{ (zero-strain)} = NH \times AF \times T$$

Thus, when we remove the hands completely from massage we transform a damaging profession into one in which practitioners can work for many years and develop excellence as practitioners. When we replace the hands with other parts of our body which can easily take the force of our body-weight, we enable practitioners to work with minimal effort and zero-strain.

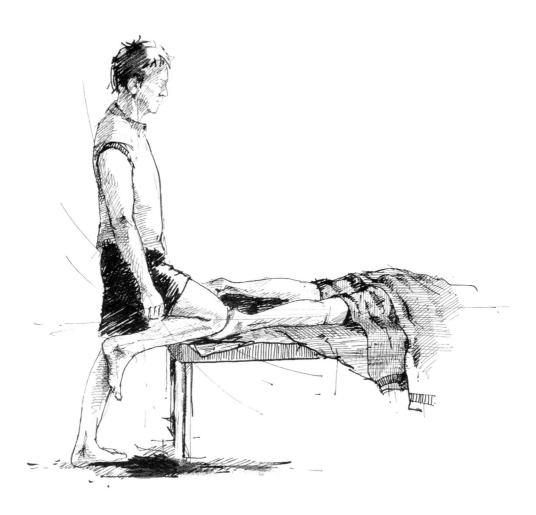

This effortless bodywork has proved itself to be an elegant approach to healing whilst also creating an increase in effectiveness. It has resulted in producing a third component into the Z-Formula, represented by the letter 'E', wherein the 'E' stands for five different meanings simultaneously:

E = Effortless

E = Energetic

E = Effective

E = Elegant

E = Excellence

or "effortlessly energetic, effective elegant excellence". We can have such 'E' bodywork *precisely because* of the zero-strain that is placed on the practitioner's body. By replacing the hands, our body-weight is now being applied over and over with parts of our body which are designed to comfortably take this level of pressure. When such techniques are performed repeatedly, there is still no increase in the risk of damage to the practitioner. This increased ability of the practitioner to work with great force or pressure with a reduction in strain results in an observable difference in the quality, energy and depth of bodywork being given.

Such an increase in potency is represented by what is now a new and winning tri-partide formula that reads:

$$Z = NHAFT = E$$

Zero-Strain =
No Hands + Applied Force + Time =
Effortless, Energetic, Effective, Elegant, Excellence

In other words, it doesn't matter how long we work or how much pressure we apply, there is no strain to the practitioner's back, hands or wrists. We have now transformed a tragically damaging equation into an equation for success for both individual bodyworkers and for the profession as a whole(1).

Short Term Gains/Long Term Losses

In the classroom where we learn traditional massage techniques, everything feels fine. When we start our practice everything looks rosy and we cannot wait to try out our new techniques and training. At this stage, traditional massage techniques are not a problem; it *is* possible to use damaging weight bearing techniques with bent wrists, or fingers and thumbs, *for a short time*.

Now, use these techniques again and again, day in and day out, over several years, and a different and damaging story emerges: fatigued, aching and troublesome thumbs, wrist and fingers. This is the real picture of the profession that I witness every day in my contact with graduates.

In addition, once we are in clinical practice, it often becomes hard to look after ourselves when faced with the pressure of time and the demands of our clients. As bodyworkers we are often driven by the needs of our clients, and our financial need to maintain and build our professional reputation. Our clients want us to be the same effective bodyworkers that we were last week.

Unfortunately clients don't appreciate us saying: "I've done this wonderful, powerful, deep and effective work on the client before you, so I'm going to give my thumbs a rest during your session.". Especially if we then add ". . . but I will still charge you the same fee.". The real price that practitioners are paying, however, is in delayed damage to their wrists and hands.

One of the problems is that as practitioners of health and healing, we do not always take the issue of looking after ourselves seriously. Often we can become hooked on the 'highs' that result from successfully looking after others. In the excitement or mood lift which can follow such a fulfilling and intimate therapy as massage, we can easily forget our own needs for self preservation.

It is not easy for massage practitioners to admit to having any health problems. Such admissions are often associated with failure. Despite the fact that it's the normal experience for most people to have some periods of illness or injury in their lives, there is still a special shame reserved for health practitioners, or healers when we are ill or damaged. After all, we're the advocates of healthy living and are meant to be the experts! The fear is that we are a bit of a 'con' if we cannot keep ourselves well.

Of the reticence of practitioners to own up to injury, Greene (1999) says:

> *"Perhaps it was just too incongruous for a healer, someone who was supposed to assuage pain in her clients, to be in pain herself... so massage professionals (and students) suffered in silence, chalked up their pain to one of the "necessary evils" of the work and just lived with it."*

This shame at being damaged is the very antithesis of healing. It is often only through being ill that we find the compassion to reach out to others and to help them. There is an unfathomable wisdom that can come with illness. For some there seems to be a profound learning inherent in every illness. For me, it was only through being ill for 18 months with ME that I learned how to reconnect with myself and my body – and as a result become a bodyworker. It was only through admitting that my wrists were in pain that I discovered this creative and expressive 'new' form of bodywork.

Another possible source of shame is that some practitioners believe they have damaged themselves because they weren't doing the massage strokes properly! Well, the good news is that you've probably done nothing wrong. The bad news is that, unfortunately - you were probably trained to injure yourself! It could be precisely because you are such a good practitioner that you are damaged.

As a result of this professional reticence to admit to injury, there has been a conspiracy of silence and a lack of dealing with the real cause of the problem, namely the use of hands in bodywork. This means that there are still many practitioners who have no damage or injury who are *carrying on using the same techniques that will injure them in the future*. If you are one of these uninjured practitioners, then I want you to read the following message three times so that you have the opportunity to protect yourself from all future damage:

> ***If your bodywork practice causes you no serious pain or injury, then now is the time to adopt zero-strain techniques so you remain a healthy practitioner.***

Those of you who have no manifesting injuries are the lucky ones - for the rest of us, No Hands Massage is simply a question of survival!

Chapter 4   Assessing your Practice

In this chapter you are invited to assess your current massage practice and to consider areas of change in technique that might be needed in order to maintain and continue developing your bodywork without risk of injury to yourself.

Assessing Your Stroke Pattern

This exercise is aimed at assessing how much of your body you are using during your bodywork. Either 'guestimate' the percentages in order to complete the Stroke Pattern Chart, below - or, even better, get together with a couple of bodywork colleagues and record the amount of time actually spent using each of the six touch categories outlined, using a stop watch. Fill in the percentage of overall massage time that you have spent using each of the different parts of your body itemised. In a typical 50 minute session, each percent represents one half of a minute:

Fig 2 Stroke Pattern Chart

1	Light Palmar Touch (whole hand techniques, but little or no pressure)	_____ %
2	Heavy Palmar Touch (using strength or body-weight applied over the whole palm and fingers)	_____ %
3	Wrist (using strength or body-weight on the base of hand - thenar and hypo thenar eminences)	_____ %
4	Fingers and Thumb (where some force is applied, as in kneading, petrissage etc)	_____ %
5	Forearm	_____ %
6	Other Body Parts	_____ %
	Total (should add up to 100%)	_____ %

Whilst this pattern may vary slightly according to the type of session given and the different needs of each client, you can quickly come to an overall average for your bodywork if you repeat this exercise a few times(1).

What Constitutes a 'Healthy Stroke Pattern'?

If your score for the Forearm (No.5) and for Other Body Parts (No.6) combined was less than 80% then the approach in this book, if followed, could prolong your massage life.

Over the years, I have compiled a 'rough average' of the stroke patterns amongst the students I have encountered. This has focused on the predominant use of the wrists, fingers and thumbs, in line with conventional approaches to training. These figures can be represented by the following statistics; they are provided so that you can compare your own stroke pattern with the average stroke pattern I encountered in the North of England:

Fig 3 Average Stroke Pattern Encountered

1	Light Palmar Touch	10%
2	Heavy Palmar Touch	15%
3	Wrist	20%
4	Fingers and Thumb	50%
5	Forearm	3%
6	Other	2%

In order to reduce self-damage, we need to increase the amount of time spent using parts of our bodies which are less susceptible to strain and injury. To achieve this, we need to decrease our use of fingers, thumbs and wrists, as well as heavy palmar work.

If we wish to eradicate any strain whatsoever from our hands (zero-strain), then we need to eliminate the Heavy Palmar Touch, the Fingers and Thumb, and the Wrist categories from our stroke profile.

Whilst 'zero-strain' sounds a logical idea that we may wish to implement immediately, in reality the following is the pattern with which I and many of my students have ended up working. It seems that when the hands are properly rested and protected, after a period of 'zero-strain' massage, then traditional techniques find a new and much reduced role in massage practice.

Fig 4 Recommended 'Practitioner Survival' Stroke Pattern

1	Light Palmar Touch	10%
2	Heavy Palmar Touch	5%
3	Wrist	5%
4	Fingers and Thumb	5%
5	Forearm	60%
6	Other	15%

The difference between what is conventional and what I am suggesting can be seen graphically through the chart, below. Look particularly at the reduction in heavy palmar work, as well as in Wrist, Fingers and Thumb use.

Fig 5 Comparison of Average Stroke Pattern and Recommended Stroke Pattern

		Stroke Pattern	
		Average	*Recommended*
1	Light Palmar Touch	10%	10%
2	Heavy Palmar Touch	15%	5%
3	Wrist	20%	5%
4	Fingers and Thumb	50%	5%
5	Forearm	3%	60%
6	Other	2%	15%

The Redundant Hand?

The recommended stroke pattern outlined in Fig 4 is the answer to the question "How can I do massage as effectively, or even more effectively, without stress to my hand or wrist?".

By removing strain from the hand, we do not seek to replace the intense sensitivity of palmar contact or the gentle reassurance that this touch can provide. The healing touch of the palm of your hand cannot be replaced by any other areas of your body. Instead, we replace the hands with forearms and other large, robust surfaces of our body for all work that involves a *high intensity of pressure*.

Translated into bodywork terms, this means that whenever doing deep, strong, heavy muscular work, we should never use our hands, and instead must look to use other body parts which can transfer our force and weight on to our clients without damage to ourselves. Whenever we do this, we honour, preserve and validate our hands and their amazing sensitivity.

To use our hands for deep and heavy structural work is an insult to such instruments of attunement and sensitivity. In my opinion, our hands are best employed in diagnosing (both structurally and intuitively), and in providing reassurance and healing contact with our clients. The hand is also the part which produces and passes on to our clients the many 'energy effects' that bodyworkers and healers have regarded as commonplace over the millennia. Scientists are still heroically struggling to measure this 'energy effect'; when they do I am sure that the centre of the palm of the hand will figure as large in their results as it does in ancient healing traditions(2).

The No Hands approach, then, is a validation and endorsement of all that your hand does best, and a protection and validation of the healer that lies within each and every bodyworker. In order to achieve this protection, we must choose alternative surfaces from the wide array of body parts available to the practitioner. For clarity, we can divide these surfaces into four zones of the body.

Chapter 5   The Four Bodywork Zones

All bodywork can be divided into the use of four zones of the practitioner's body, which I call the Primary, Secondary, Tertiary, and Quarterly zones.

The *primary zone* consists of any part of the body from the wrist to the tips of the fingers (distal to the wrist joint). The *secondary zone* consists of any part between the elbow and the wrist joint of the forearm (distal to the elbow); this basically means the forearm. The *tertiary zone* consists of any part of the upper arm (distal to the shoulder joint), and the *quarterly zone* consists of any other parts of the body, namely torso, head, legs and feet.

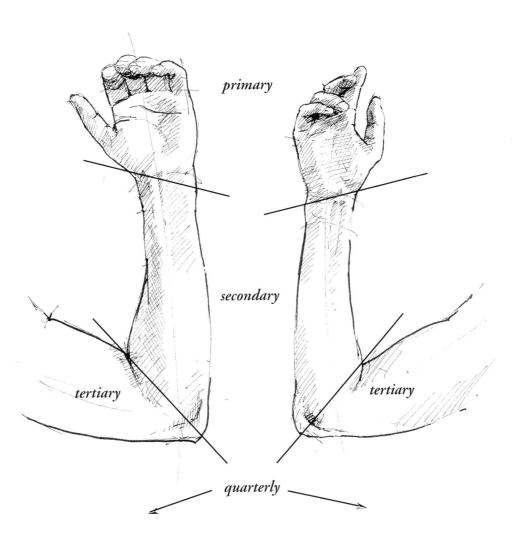

primary

secondary

tertiary   *tertiary*

quarterly

1   The Primary Zone

THE HAND

The hands are used in a way which minimises damage to the practitioner and maximises the sensitivity and 'gazelle-like' nature of the hand. All light stroking and holding techniques use the hand for what it is best at: palpation, diagnosis, intuition, and energetic rebalancing work.

2   The Secondary Zone

THE FOREARM

The forearm is the mainstay of the No Hands Massage approach, and provides a wide variety of surfaces and options for effective, effortless and creative bodywork, utilising the strong 'shire horse' aspect of the forearms.

3   The Tertiary Zone

THE UPPER ARM

This is rarely used on its own, but provides a powerful surface for full body-weight techniques.

4   The Quarterly Zone

THE REST OF THE BODY

Sometimes the legs and the knees and the feet can be utilised for highly efficient bodywork movements.

Chapter 6   The Forearm – Seven Surfaces

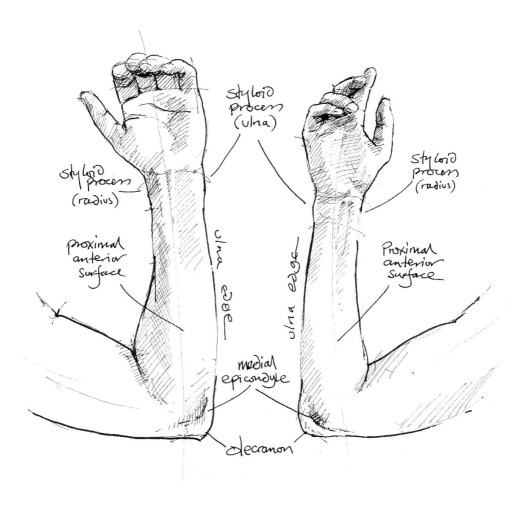

styloid process (ulna)

styloid process (radius)

styloid process (radius)

proximal anterior surface

Proximal anterior surface

ulna edge

ulna edge

medial epicondyle

olecranon

1   The Soft Front   (proximal, anterior surface of forearm)

This is the soft and pliable part of the forearm. The softer part is fatty tissue closest to the elbow. This is where most of the work is done. This part quite adequately replaces soft, medium and heavy palmar effleurage and can work most muscle groups of the body. In many ways the soft tissue of this part of the forearm provides more possibilities than does the palm, as it 'moulds' and 'gives' more easily to whatever part of our client's body we are applying pressure. It thus responds to the contours of the client's body in a way that is different and sometimes more effective than the palm.

Self Practise Exercise 1   The Soft Front

Feel down this surface of your arm. Now press the soft tissue of the front of your forearm against a variety of surfaces, the edge of your chair, a table and notice how well it moulds, like water, around any object with which it comes into contact.

The front forearm's softness and the greater surface area (it is a bigger 'pad' than the palm), make it possible to apply much more body-weight without any discomfort to our client. This makes for some very pleasant passive stretching, in which the stroke simultaneously both effleurages and stretches the muscle, encouraging it to lengthen without any effort or pain.

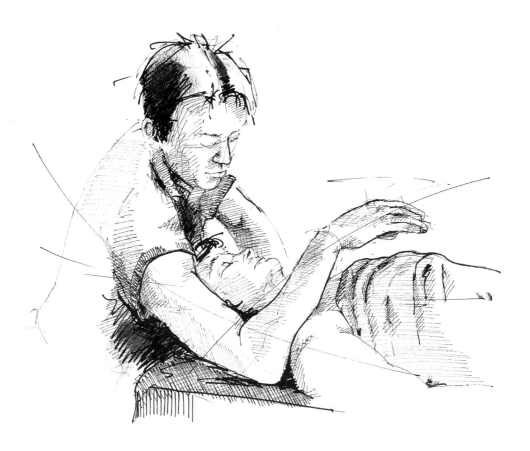

Psychological impact

The psychological impact of such a powerful combination of compression, effleurage and passive stretching is often one of release and letting go *of the whole body*, no matter which part of the body is worked on. This soft front is the zone of your body that you work with most in No Hands Massage. It is the safest part to use (providing the seven postural principles are adhered to) whilst your brain builds up a new 'sensitivity database' from the movements you are making.

When using this soft part of the forearm, your brain adjusts to 'reading' the information that the nerves from this part of your body are sending you, as well as the different information you are gathering from all your senses and the rest of your body. After a while it becomes possible to pick up your client's subtle responses to your work as effectively through the forearms as through the palms - it just takes a while to make the transition. As that transition becomes complete, it is safe to work with some of the other, less soft, surfaces of your body.

2   The Hard Back

This is the harder posterior surface of the forearm. It has less fatty tissue and more muscle than the anterior surface. As a consequence it is less pliable.

> *Self Practise Exercise 2   The Hard Back*
>
> *Feel down this surface of your arm. Now press the soft tissue of the back of your forearm against a variety of surfaces, the edge of your chair, a table and notice how little 'give' there is to any object with which it comes into contact. Compare it with your soft front by leaning into your thigh, first with the front and then with the back.*

The hard back can be used for firmer and deeper work. The bones of both the radius and the ulna can be felt beneath its surface. This means that the proximal half of this posterior surface becomes harder and sharper, ending in a well-defined ulnar edge at the point of the elbow (the olecranon). Combined with the relative lack of fatty tissue, this provides the firmness for deeper petrissage and friction work. The hard back surface is useful for working at right angles to the grain of muscle-fibres, and for applying deeper and more circular movements. More specific compressions become possible and the hard back is extremely effective in the application of neuro-muscular techniques. *Extra care must be taken when using this part of the body, so as not to cause discomfort or pain to the client.*

3   The Point

This is the point at the tip of your elbow (the olecranon).

This is a wonderful replacement for the thumb in the application of compression and friction techniques, acupressure point work, and trigger point work. As it has fewer sensory nerves than the thumb, maximum care needs to be taken in the placement of this point on the body. It also needs careful support from the other hand, to avoid any danger of slipping across and bruising the clients tissues, and to provide sensory feedback from the surrounding tissues. This support, safety and feedback is most easily provided by laying the non-working hand flat on the body and applying the point in the right angle of the web between thumb and forefinger.

> *Self Practise Exercise 3   The Point*
>
> *To experiment with this, place the palm of your left hand face down on your thigh, forming a right angle between your thumb and forefinger. Now press into the thigh with the point of your right arm, making sure that your right elbow is pushed snugly into this right angle. In this position it becomes possible to put considerable, but controlled pressure on to muscle knots and trigger points, and to make small rotations and vibrational movements that are effective for many types of soft-tissue work.*

The support hand also becomes a support arm, in that the whole arm can often be laid flat on the client's body. This means you can comfortably lean your weight on to this flat arm thereby taking the strain from your back (see Postural Principle 'Triangulation'). The result is a posturally secure and sensory rich technique.

4   The Ulnar Edge

This is the part of your arm that faces the floor as you do a karate chop downwards.

> *Self Practise Exercise 4   The Ulnar Edge*
>
> *Hold the base of your forearm, just above the elbow. Now rotate your wrist each way and feel how the edge can be more or less exposed. In the*

anatomical position, when you rotate your wrist laterally it brings the soft
tissue on the posterior surface alongside the bone, and when you rotate your
wrist medially it brings the soft tissue of the anterior surface of your forearm
alongside the ridge, in both cases making the ridge less sharp.

This is a hard, sharp edge that can be drawn across the muscle fibres of the body, as if "sawing wood". It adequately replaces the base of the wrist and the thumbs for a variety of deep techniques. The amount of this edge you use whilst applying downward pressure dictates the depth of specific 'cut' you are making into the tissues of the body. The more of a friction type stroke you want, the more edge you use. Rotating your wrist during the sawing motion alters the amount of sawing edge that is active. Identifying just how much 'cut' your client can take, without experiencing discomfort, is probably the most important sensitivity in using this surface.

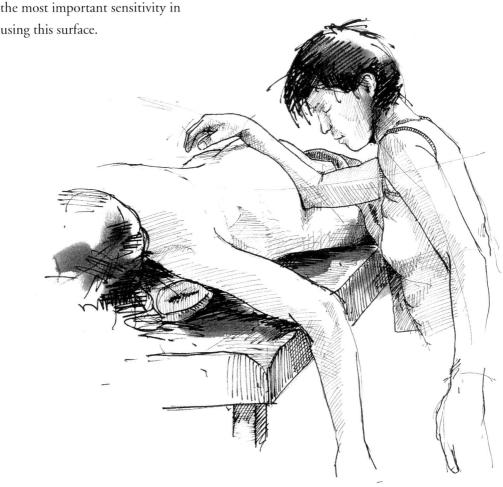

5   The Soft Point

This is the small bone just on the inside of the elbow joint (medial epicondyle of humerus). With the arm outstretched in the anatomical position, it is the bone next to the body, whilst the olecranon is posterior. Colloquially known as the *funny bone*.

This is another point which can be utilised, particularly when applying sideways pressure to the client's body.

> *Self Practise Exercise 5   The Soft Point*
>
> *Bend your arm to form a right angle, with your hand pointing up to the ceiling. Now bring your arm across the front of your body twisting your wrist (palm turning towards your face) as you go. This is a traditional Karate 'block' movement. As you make the end of this movement you bring the epicondyle into play. You can place your other hand on this soft point as you do the movement.*

This little bone provides a useful hook with which to apply stretches to various parts of the body, as well as providing a useful point that can be used for deeper structural strokes.

Care must be taken of the practitioner's own body, as the ulna nerve passes close to this surface, hence the 'funny bone' syndrome. However it is a very useful point to apply at the end of some movements, and provides a sharper point for deeper work.

6   The V

This is the angle of forearm and upper arm. I call it the V because the bones are in the shape of a V. This technique uses both secondary and tertiary zones of the body.

The V is achieved by fully flexing your arm so the wrist is as close to your shoulder as is comfortable. Both the posterior and the anterior surfaces become available for different types of work or pressure. It provides a very large pad indeed for the application of much pressure, whichever way it is used.

Self Practise Exercise 6   The V

Form a V as described above. Feel the large pad that this V creates about 4 inches above and below the elbow when your hand comes as close to your shoulder as possible. Feel both posterior and anterior surfaces of this V. These are very useful pads for any movements which involve the practitioner in applying leaning pressure against or away from the client. Now, find a door jamb. Holding your arm in this V position, across your chest, push your body away from the doorway. You should be able to apply this technique to easily move your whole body-weight.

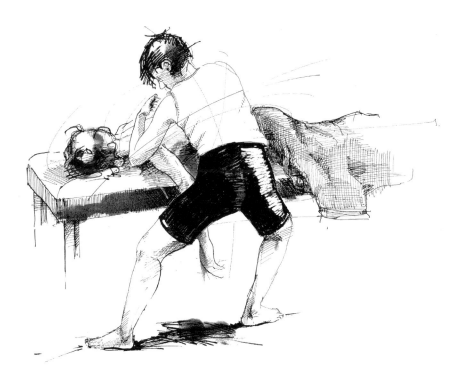

What this exercise shows is how effortlessly we can apply *our whole body-weight* during bodywork without any damage to ourselves or to our client.

The posterior surface can be used for a whole-body push, rather as in pushing into a rugby scrum. In addition, the anterior surface of the V can be used for a whole-body pull or lean, rather like leaning away from a lamp post.

7   The Small Hooks

These can be found at the distal ends of the radius and ulna bones.

These are useful little edges which can be increased or decreased in size by changing the position of the wrist. Their effectiveness can be reduced or increased by the amount of body-weight applied behind them.

Self Practise Exercise 7   The Small Hooks

Place one wrist on top of the other in front of you. Push these edges against each other, applying reasonable pressure. The Radial (top) ridge of your lower arm should be hooking into the ulnar (bottom) edge of your upper arm. Experiment with ways to get a good firm hook on each arm.

These hooks can be useful in applying powerful techniques in places where the much larger forearm cannot fit.

Conclusion

As can be seen from these seven surfaces, massage practitioners have at their disposal a veritable warehouse of tools from which to select the appropriate massage movements. I would like to stress that all the parts of the arm shown in this chapter as bodywork tools need to be used with the seven postural principles outlined in the rest of this book in order to be both safe and effective for the practitioner and client alike.

自然

PART 2　　SEVEN POSTURAL PRINCIPLES

Introduction

This introductory section gives two self-exploratory exercises which can be practised before reading the seven chapters on the seven postural principles which I have identified.

Physical beginnings

Where precisely does a massage stroke begin? The answer to this question should direct all our thoughts about posture and movement during bodywork, yet this fundamental question does not often seem to be given the attention it deserves in bodywork literature.

If we are to believe bodywork diagrams and pictures with their emphasis on hand techniques, then the answer is a simple one: a massage stroke begins in the hands, followed by movement in the shoulders, followed by movement in the rest of the body. This is absurd.

To answer the question "Where does the movement for each stroke begin?", we need to explore all our body movements. The answers we come up with will be relevant to all bodyworkers, from beauticians to osteopaths. The following exercise will help you to explore this issue.

Self Practise Exercise 8   Physical Beginnings

Stand in the middle of the room, with your knees slightly bent and close your eyes so that you activate your kinaesthetic awareness. Do this by noticing the physical sensations of your breathing, and the contact of your feet against the floor. Spend at least 10 breaths getting yourself connected with your body and your physical sensations.

Remember to make sure that your knees are slightly bent. By shutting your eyes and cutting out visual stimuli, by stilling your thinking mind and by focusing on your breath and feet, you will strengthen your awareness of physical sensations, thereby developing kinaesthetic awareness. It is this kinaesthetic awareness that will guide our postural ruminations.

Think of a massage stroke you know well, and use often. Begin making the movements of this stroke in slow motion, taking at least twice as long as normal. Do this several times. Now, concentrate on the first third of this stroke. What movements within your body are you noticing at the beginning of the stroke?

Slowing down even further, as if stretching time itself, make this first part of the stroke last 10 seconds. This means you are moving at a twentieth of the speed as when massaging your clients. Your brain has the opportunity to notice twenty times as much about your movements. What do you notice about the beginning of your favourite stroke?

Where do the movements begin in your body? Which part of you moves first? Make a mental note of your findings. Now begin this stroke by first moving from different parts of your body. Try your arms, try your feet, try your hips, your belly and your knees. See what actually fits your own internal experiences best.

Before reading on, keep doing this until you come up with your own thoughts and sensations about the beginning of each stroke.

Annotate your findings about the origins of your movements - you may have several different thoughts at this stage. Spend as long as you want on this, and ask this question during each bodywork session: "Where in my body do I begin each stroke?". What I am suggesting is that you discard all taught theories and simply feel for the beginnings of each physical movement within your own body.

Energetic beginnings

Now, we will feel for the energetic beginnings of each stroke. These are the energy movements, or the stirrings of that 'pre-physical movement' within the body, just prior to the actual movement. I invite you to explore these energetic beginnings of each movement just prior to your actual physical movements.

Self Practise Exercise 9   Energetic Beginnings

Now do the same exercise as above. Close your eyes, bend your knees and connect once again to the physical sensations of your breath and your 'kinaesthetic awareness'.

This time, before you actually make the movements of your massage stroke, feel for the impulse of energy within your being that precedes each actual movement. Do several strokes, each time starting from stillness, and feeling for the 'pre-stroke' stirrings within you.

Do this for several strokes. Where do you feel the impulse for each movement beginning? When you think you have it, then imagine this impulse emanating from different parts of your body. Feel for where in your body best fits your own experience of this initial impulse towards movement, just prior to the movement itself, and make a mental note of your experiences.

Do both of these exercises several times and annotate your thoughts and answers each time before reading on. Whatever anyone else tells you about posture is less important than what you actually experience and become aware of for yourself. This is why it is valuable to take a break before reading further, in order to spend time experimenting with these exercises. It is best if you experiment with the exercises during your bodywork sessions over the next few weeks. Time spent doing this will enhance your appreciation and understanding of the following pages, as well as develop your self awareness as a practitioner.

The seven postural principles

The following chapters identify the seven postural principles which underpin No Hands Massage. For each postural principle covered, an exercise is offered which demonstrates the principle. In Part 3 of this book, seven zero-strain massage strokes are shown, and the relevant postural principles are discussed for each stroke.

Chapter 7   Postural Principle One

Begin in the Belly

I believe that all massage strokes begin energetically in the practitioner's belly. This is also called *the Hara* in oriental literature. If you found anything different during your experiments using the previous exercises, then I invite you to keep an open mind during this chapter, and if what I write does not fit for you, then discard it at the end. What matters is your experience of movement, regardless of what anyone else, including me, tells you.

Before anything actually moves there is an impulse, an activation towards movement, a stirring in the belly. According to shiatsu principles, practically all our Meridians and energy lines emanate outwards from this 'centre', radiating out to the limbs and returning back again. Masters of Shiatsu can diagnose and treat the energy imbalances of the whole body through the belly. Masunaga (1987)

The Hara is the place from which we drew our nourishment and our life force in the womb. The Hara is the place into which we breathe and from which we breathe out. As the seat of this life force, Buddha figures are shown with wonderfully rounded bellies. Unlike our modern day fetish about trim torsos, the large belly was regarded as a sign of wisdom and power in oriental art and literature.

Self Practise Exercise 10   Breathing the Belly

Stand in the middle of your room with your legs slightly apart and your knees bent. Place your hands on your belly. Feel your breath entering and leaving your belly. Let your belly expand with each in-breath, and collapse with each exhalation. Close your eyes as you do this. Open up your kinaesthetic awareness to all the physical sensations of your standing and your breathing. Make this the centre of your focus, your belly, your breath, your connectedness.

This is Hara awareness. Do this for several minutes, each breath entering and leaving your belly unhurriedly. Breathe in through your nose and out through your open mouth. Let the sound of your outbreath be a "downward" sound, the sound of "HAW". With each breath, let your weight sink further into the ground. Feel yourself growing stronger and more powerful with each breath.

Now, keeping your eyes shut, begin to walk slowly about the room; only do this from your belly. Let each movement and change of direction come from your belly. Lead with your belly. Keep your knees bent, your body-weight low and your movements very, very slow. Now you are moving and breathing from your belly.

Notice how you feel after doing this for just a few minutes.

Now, go back to *Self Practise Exercise 9 Energetic Beginning*s, on page 46, and this time let your belly create the impulse for each movement. Let each stroke emanate from your belly.

Chapter 8   Postural Principle Two

It's All in the Sole

Following its energetic beginning in the belly, I believe that the stroke movement is immediately followed by a 'dropping down' of the practitioner's body-weight into the feet, giving an almost instantaneous grounding. Without this 'anchoring', our movements can lack potency or power.

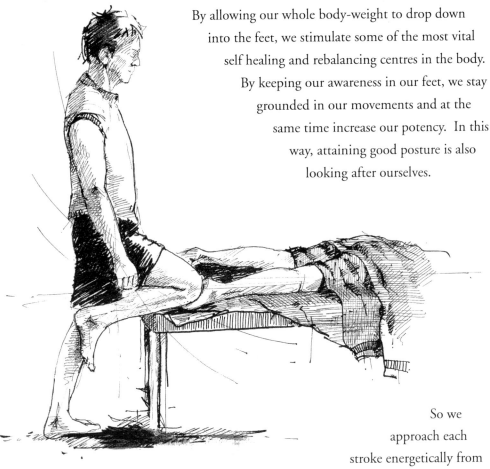

By allowing our whole body-weight to drop down into the feet, we stimulate some of the most vital self healing and rebalancing centres in the body. By keeping our awareness in our feet, we stay grounded in our movements and at the same time increase our potency. In this way, attaining good posture is also looking after ourselves.

So we approach each stroke energetically from the Hara, our 'belly-centre', and then allow it to drop down into our feet. This is accompanied by an actual physical lowering of our

Stand in the middle of the room, legs apart, keeping your knees bent, breathing into your belly. Do this for several breaths. Good. Now let the weight of your belly drop down into your feet. Do this by letting your lower back lengthen, tucking your pelvis slightly under. Accompany this with a slight lowering of your knees. Make this a very small movement. Make sure your upper body stays upright and your chest nice and open and wide. Focus your mind's attention on the soles of your feet. Can you feel that 'dropping down' in your feet? Repeat this several times, letting yourself experience the intensification of awareness in your feet, as you let your body-weight drop down into your soles.

Now that you are feeling the soles of your feet, start making small movements with your belly, keeping your feet stationary on the ground. Notice how each movement is experienced in the sole of your foot. By slowly moving your belly to different places you can activate different reflexes in your foot. By moving your belly and torso slowly, you can feel the different reflex zones of your foot becoming activated. Imagine that someone is actually massaging your foot through the floor. This 'self-reflexology' is a pleasant rebalancing exercise that you can do almost anywhere, at any time. Do this for as long as you wish - even a minute will be beneficial, and 5-10 minutes will awaken and energise all the reflexes in your foot for the day.

Now, let yourself be still, and make the same massage movement that you chose for Self Practice Exercise 8. This time drop your awareness into your belly. Drop your weight into your feet and now let the soles of your feet push down into the ground as you make your massage stroke movement. Remember, belly, feet, movement. Feel every movement you make on this floor-foot interface. Imagine that you are directing this massage through the soles of your feet.

Again, notice how you feel after spending time getting connected with your feet. This is a powerful self-healing exercise as it stimulates and awakens reflexes throughout your whole foot, and this in turn can stimulate your own self-healing.

The purpose of these movements is to show how No Hands Massage is really a whole body movement form. Any change of direction or force is produced, not by the muscles of the upper arm and body, but by the belly, hips and legs of the practitioner. These movements can be felt most clearly in the changes of pressure and torque in the soles of the feet.

Empowering your massage

When we attain this connection with our feet, and experience each massage movement as emanating from our feet, then all our massage strokes will have power and energy. It is from this 'Earth-element', this ancient root, that all our bodywork movements spring up, through our legs and torso, into the arms and finally, into the hands or arms. It is from this Earth that we draw up the energy necessary to help others, without exhausting and depleting ourselves. Without dropping our weight from the belly into our feet, into the Earth, and letting this powerful elemental force of nature power our movements, we are disempowering both ourselves and our bodywork.

Awareness and massage injury

From the sole of the foot, each massage movement we make travels upwards and outwards culminating in contact with the client's body. Bodyworkers who can feel each movement they make in the soles of their feet are so attuned and self-aware *that it is virtually impossible to do harm either to themselves or to their clients.*

Bigger muscles make the movement

Because the practitioner is rooted in the ground, the force and strain of these strokes is taken up by the strong and structurally less vulnerable muscles of the lower body. From the gluteals downwards, these lower body muscles are working many times harder than in conventional massage postures. As a result, many erstwhile sacrosanct postural rules can now be broken. Instead of the sometimes rather wobbly leaning tower of Pisa that I witness in conventional massage strokes, we now have a powerful pyramid, a far stronger support structure which will stand the test of time without the need for any scaffolding.

Chapter 9   Postural Principle Three

Flow

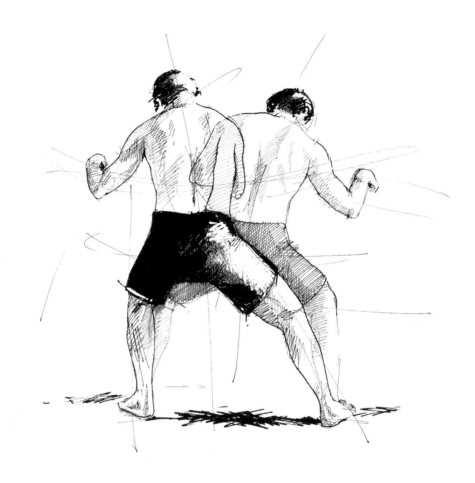

The problem of 'proper posture'

Much postural theory in bodywork literature is presented through necessarily stiff and static drawings or photographs which portray the angles and lines of so-called 'proper stance'. These images, which we hold in our heads whilst working, can influence the way we move when doing bodywork. Such static lines and angles are detrimental to the bodyworker. Rigid angular images in massage books are likely to produce rigid body movements in the practitioner. What we need instead are more poetic ways of describing posture(1).

Dynamic imagery

The human body was never designed to be static. Because of this, I prefer to use the dynamic language of primal and elemental imagery to capture what I believe are the core principles of bodywork posture. So far, I have used the element Earth and words such as 'rooted', 'anchored' and 'grounded' to convey the postural principles for 'belly' and 'feet'.

For the third postural principle then, we need to hold in our minds the dynamic image conjured up by the word 'FLOW'. To evoke this postural principle, I encourage practitioners to think in terms of the element *Water* and the concept of 'whole body flow'. To do this, I invite you to try the following exercise.

Self Practise Exercise 12   Water Movement

Put on a piece of serene, tranquil, flowing music. (It is worth noting that music with the sound of the sea may not always be the best choice.) Standing in the middle of the room, with knees bent and eyes shut activate your kinaesthetic awareness of your breath, your belly and your feet. Spend a few breaths doing this.

Gently sway from side to side, and then forwards and backwards. Let your arms enter into this swaying and flowing. Let the sound of your breath be part of this ebbing and flowing movement. Keep your body movements grounded by dropping your weight into the ground and flowing from your feet. Imagine each movement you make to be dropping down to the Earth (like rain) and then flowing powerfully forwards like the sea. Let your arms be the movements of a Tai Chi master.

Now imagine you are in your massage room, giving a 'water massage'. Imagine yourself slowly moving around the table and massaging with your whole body movements - as if the client could feel all your movements as well as the strokes. Feel all your movements flow from your belly, down into your feet and then up through your legs into the rest of your body.

If this relaxing and self-healing exercise is done just a few times to the same piece of music, then simply playing this music during your next bodywork session will programme your body to flow more during the session(2).

This exercise is about experiencing the sensations of water flowing back and forth within our bodies, as water flows against the shore then back to the ocean. When applied to a bodywork session, it is about the practitioner's body becoming the flowing element of water *throughout the session*. This elemental approach, with its variety of moods and temperaments provides the practitioner with a wide range of options for bodywork strokes. Water can be stormy and wild, as well as calm and soothing.

If we hold such flowing elemental images in our minds during bodywork sessions, then we are less likely to damage our bodies. Such images have to be an improvement on the constricted and stiff movements shown in the conventional and rather rigid drawings of so-called 'correct posture'. When flowing elemental images replace thoughts about "getting the correct posture", practitioner creativity also increases.

Thus, I am less interested in the rigidity of holding the "correct posture", than in the constant changing of position, the ebb and flow of movements made during a bodywork session. I believe that only when such fluidity of movement is present can we be said to be truly protecting ourselves with good posture.

As you allow your body to flow, your muscles contract and relax. With such ever-changing posture, sustained and damaging tensions will struggle to find a home anywhere in your body. The postures that accompany such elemental movements are therefore *all* 'correct'. Flow creates ease and this creates pleasure, self healing and creativity for the practitioner.

Massage as dance

The human body is designed to be able to take up all sorts of beautiful, weird and wonderful postures. Let us not limit ourselves by any rigid line-drawn rule books. What is damaging to the practitioner's own body is held and constricted positions (whether 'posturally correct' or not). What is healing for the practitioner's body is to constantly change and move and flow. Tai Chi is an impressive example of the healing power that flowing and graceful movements can have. I also believe that these flowing movements can have beneficial effects on the client when they become an integral part of each bodywork session(3). The oriental discipline of Chi Kung also holds that the whole body movements of a practitioner can have beneficial results for the client(4).

54

The human bodyworker, then, is a dancer who is in continuous movement, creating his own physical poetry. To watch such a bodyworker is to be mesmerised by flow and movement and by the beauty and grace of such an elemental bodywork form. For this reason, I am more concerned with the interactions between all the different muscle groups of the practitioner *as a whole*, than in simplistic vectors of physics.

I find learning about this poetry of motion and its ensuing 'stillnesses' far more useful than learning about the science of "proper posture". It is this poetic motion that I encourage in my bodywork students with the postural language of elemental imagery. Such elemental language helps to characterise the speed and force with which bodywork is given. Such a focus on the type of movements produced in *the bodyworker's own body*, produces a quantum shift in the quality of massage given, and puts training effective bodyworkers into the same realm as training dancers.

One massage stroke per session

To experience the power of this flow principle, we do all the things which are normally considered "not massage" as part of the massage. In conventional massage, the majority of massage strokes are most often defined by contact with the client's skin. In No Hands Massage the massage stroke is defined as beginning at the start of the session as the practitioner closes the door and moves towards the client lying on the table, and ends as the practitioner closes the door at the end of the session.

What this means is that, even when draping the client or applying oil to our hands, we remain in the flowing movement of the watery massage. Even when in apparent 'stillness', when our hands and bodies appear still, we can experience the continual movement of energy within our own bodies. This is often experienced as 'currents in the sea', or as 'spirals within the body'. With practise, such subtle movements can even be felt by the practitioner from within the client's body.

Self Practise Exercise 13   The Flow of Stillness

To experience the inner flow of energy - the so called 'stillness' – repeat Self Practice Exercise 12. After a few minutes of these flowing movements, lie down on the floor and feel the movements continuing in your body. Don't worry if you don't feel this at first, keep doing this exercise daily until you do.

At first, if you can't feel them, just pretend you can. Imagine currents within your body moving between your head and your feet and from side to side and from the back of your body to the front. Imagine all these currents meeting, intermingling, and spiralling throughout your body. Soon you will not need to imagine it, you will be experiencing such currents of energy, physically.

Once we attune ourselves to an awareness of subtle energetic movements within ourselves, we soon begin to feel such movements within our clients(5). Once we employ an awareness of flow in our sessions, without necessarily knowing why or realising what is going on that is different, clients often report a deepening of the massage and an increase in the effect of the massage on body and mind.

Chapter 10   Postural Principle Four

Falling Over Massage

This is what we do during No Hands Massage, we lean on our client by falling over gracefully on to them. . . more of a lean than a push. If we push we strain, use our muscles and tire. If we lean, as against a counter, we transfer our weight with awareness on to our client, creating a powerful and sensitive pressure. If we literally 'fell' on to our client then this would cause them pain. It is more of a slow motion transfer of our weight from the ground on to our client, as described in my introduction.

Transferring weight

When working on a client, our body-weight is normally distributed in varying proportions on to the four points of our two feet and our two hands. This four point contact means that bodywork is more akin to crawling or climbing than it is to upright walking. This is an important consideration when discussing stance. To walk without strain is a very different proposition to crawling without strain. Most of this chapter is about how to crawl, as that is what bodywork is really about. In order to lean well, we need to learn to crawl like babies.

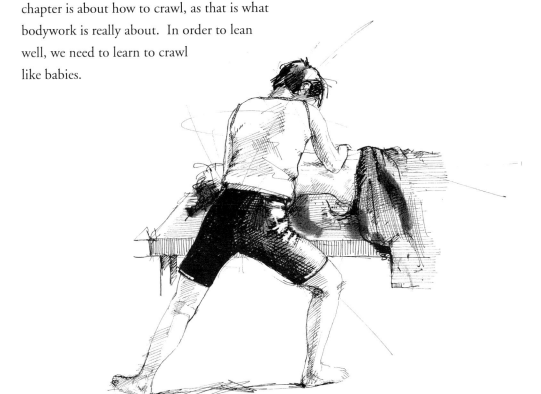

Self Practise Exercise 14   Crawling Bodywork

In the middle of the room, place yourself on all fours in a crawling position. Feel the weight distribution on your knees and hands. Slowly move from side to side, forwards and backwards, imagining yourself 'filling' the arm or leg on to which you are transferring your weight, and emptying the arm or leg from which you are taking weight away. Breathe into your belly and let your belly hang down with the force of gravity. See how slowly you can move your weight from one arm or leg to another arm or leg. You are now experiencing transference of weight.

When working in traditional western bodywork style using a fairly high table, most of the focus of bodywork is on what is happening with the hands. Much of the practitioner's body-weight is carried by the feet - with the shoulders, arms and upper body strength employed in making the actual bodywork movements.

In No Hands Massage, the shift in weight distribution is seen as a vital part of the bodyworker's technique. This is experienced as a constant ebbing and flowing between feet and arms. It is this transference of weight which produces the sensation of leaning or "falling over" on to our client.

Self Practise Exercise 15   Leaning Bodywork

Stand facing a wall, and place your hands lightly, chest height, against the wall with all your weight going down into your feet. Now slowly lean into the wall and feel your arms filling and an increase of pressure against the wall. Then bend your knees and let the weight empty out of your arms back into your legs. See how slowly you can do this and how subtle the transfer of weight can feel. Move further away from the wall, or closer in, to experiment with different amounts of body-weight.

Self Practise Exercise 16   Falling Over Bodywork

Stand close to a plinth or table with knees bent, arms loose and your pelvis 'tucked under'. Slowly bring your forearms on to the surface of the table and transfer your weight into your hands, filling your arms and emptying your legs, as in the crawling exercise. How much and how slowly can you transfer your weight into different arms or legs?

Back strain

As bodyworkers, we can only "walk our talk" by eliminating any damage to ourselves whilst working on clients. Back strain comes from leaning forward and holding ourselves from falling. There is no need to do this in No Hands Massage. It is now safe to fall.

There is no need for excessive back tension as the practitioner falls on to their forearms; the client's body is providing support for the back. This is a tough one for many bodyworkers as it involves *letting our client support us*. It actually reflects the reality of the client-practitioner relationship. Our client supports us by feeding us, paying for our mortgages and, equally important, empowering us to grow in our own healing and awareness by lying on that plinth, playing 'client' and letting us play 'therapist'.

Form versus psychology

The key to this 'falling over' principle is to be mindful of the weight transference between feet and hands, and to move slowly. By concentrating exclusively on the *form* of your bodywork, namely the speed and amount of weight you transfer, and which surface of your own body you are using to make physical contact with your client, you will provide a safe non-invasive bodywork space that your client can fill and expand into. For myself, I do not worry about what is going on inside my client's head, I concern myself exclusively on the *form* of No Hands movements that I am making.

Whilst there is plenty of psychological or emotional information I may pick up or notice about my client, like a dancer, I channel this awareness back into the form of my massage movements. This means focusing back into my breath, my feet, my belly and my contact with the floor. This actually increases my somatic awareness of my client. The more I focus on the physical form of my work, the more I activate my own kinaesthetic senses. As I become more kinaesthetically aware I pick up more somatic information about my client's state at this moment, and the more I can address their condition through my physical, somatic work. This ensures I do what I am trained to do, namely physical work, even though the impact of what I do may have far reaching mental, emotional and even spiritual effects for my client. The client may or may not choose to inform me of these.

By focusing on the form and structure of your own movements, any energy drain that comes from becoming too immersed in your client's thought patterns can be avoided. This is one of my key principles of practitioner survival.

If you let yourself become too immersed in your client's thinking and psychology, you can get drawn into a world that does not belong to you. As you let your own mental boundaries thus merge and intermingle with those of your client, you will find yourself becoming tired more easily.

The paradox of No Hands Massage is that clearer mental boundaries can be maintained through focus on your own body movements (the *form*), even though you are physically closer and more connected to your client. This will keep you working as a bodyworker, providing therapy through physical work, and stop you turning into a psychotherapist or counsellor providing therapy through mental or verbal work.

Chapter 11   Postural Principle Five

Supported Massage

By leaning and falling over on to our clients we move into the realm of working with the principle of supported massage. What this means in a "nuts and bolts" context is that we are behaving in a very different way from conventional bodywork culture. In 'Verticality', I explore how we can support ourselves better, in 'Triangulation' I explore how we can physically let our client and the floor support us more, and in 'Secret Levers' I describe ways in which we can use the table in a supportive way.

VERTICALITY

Sitting posture

The core concept, here, is that when the back is vertical there is no strain on the bodyworker. I call this the principle of Verticality. All body-weight is transferred down into the ground, and the back muscles are doing what they are designed to do best - adjust posture and balance. If the back is called upon to lean forward for more than short periods of time, then we are placing abnormal stresses on all the joints and soft tissues of the back - with resulting micro-traumas and long term injury. Giving effective bodywork to clients with only a vertical back is very limiting, if not an impossibility. In my experience of observing bodyworkers, our backs rarely stay vertical for long.

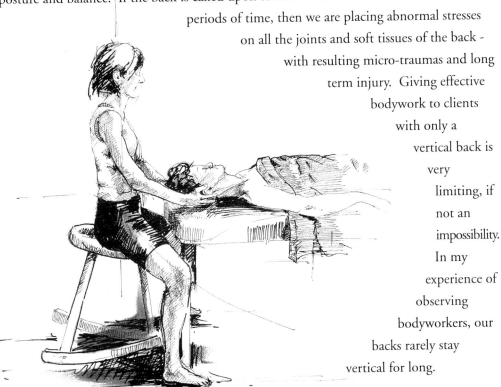

Low-force techniques

The only vertical-back strokes that are possible without damaging strain to the wrists and fingers are those done with no weight. These, by definition are light touch techniques performed on those parts of the client's body close to the practitioner's standing body, or techniques done with the practitioner sitting. When the practitioner is massaging with a vertical back, it is important to transfer weight comfortably into the ground. This is done, when sitting, through letting our upper body-weight transfer into the ground through sitting firmly on our ischeal tuberosities or 'sitz bones'

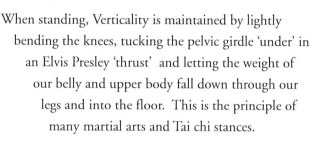

When standing, Verticality is maintained by lightly bending the knees, tucking the pelvic girdle 'under' in an Elvis Presley 'thrust' and letting the weight of our belly and upper body fall down through our legs and into the floor. This is the principle of many martial arts and Tai chi stances.

When done with awareness such 'low-force', vertical stances can be experienced by the client as extremely powerful. If our own body-weight is transferred down the spine, down through bent knees into the heels, and we are breathing into our belly, then such work - when still or gentle - can produce profoundly significant experiences for the client. The comfort and ease of the practitioner in this stance will enhance the effectiveness of whatever subtle techniques are employed.

Such a 'vertical back' approach is well documented in those massage writings that spend time on the theory of posture(1). In actual massage practice, however, even if practitioners do keep their back vertical then anytime these vertical back strokes are done with force, the muscles of the arms, shoulder girdle and upper torso are all involved in ways which create abnormal loading for the upper body. Mostly, increased force is achieved by a forward lean and the transference of weight on to the client's body. As soon as there is any transference of weight or force on to the client, or the bodyworker extends their upper arms away from vertical, then the realm of leaning is entered into.

Back strain

The practitioner's upper body-weight cannot simply disappear into the ether. No harm to the practitioner's body can be guaranteed only if the spine is kept vertical. With the spine vertical, the practitioner's weight is transferred down to the floor. In this scenario, however, we cannot work with any pressure, nor can we reach out and extend our upper arms from a vertical position. As soon as our upper arms move away from our torso we begin applying pressure and leaning, and our back muscles are brought into play. Explore this for yourself:

Self Practise Exercise 17   Arm

Standing beside your plinth - or any table equivalent to the height of your massage table - bend your knees and 'tuck' your pelvis slightly under to attain a well grounded and comfortable standing posture. Keep your hands close to your body so that your upper arms remain vertical. Experience the comfort and balance of this posture. Take several breaths and awaken your kinaesthetic awareness. Now, very slowly move your hands away from your body, towards an imaginary body on the couch - so slowly that your mind can monitor all the muscles in your own body as you do this. How far can you move your upper arms away from your body, before you become aware of the muscles down your spine becoming active?

This exercise, surprisingly, showed me that we cannot move our upper arms away from vertical without involving the whole of the spine. As soon as the upper arms move away from the torso, the back muscles contract and start 'pulling the back away' as a counterweight to the weight of the arms. This involves no visible movement in the spine, but can be experienced kinaesthetically.

Dealing with leaning

Without lean there is no weight or pressure to your bodywork. Without weight or pressure to your bodywork, there can be no massage relief to the tissues of your client's body. In other words, *there is no effective massage of the soft tissues without lean.* The paradox, then, is that in order to achieve the powerful benefits of conventional massage (of which I believe I am one of the strongest advocates) we need to abandon using our hands.

Once we do this, our forearms create total support for the spine without any damage to our hands. When employing the principles of No Hands Massage, the problem of damage to our backs, wrists and fingers is solved all in one go. Provided we do this leaning correctly, then the spine is protected through the principles of triangulation and secret levers.

TRIANGULATION

When we lean on to our client, we transfer strain from our backs on to the floor through the use of the principle of triangulation. The triangle is the strongest structure known to man. This is how we first built long bridges. The reason for this is that pressure down any one vector is dissipated across the other two in a circle of tension and strength.

Inherent in 'falling over' massage, then, is this principle of triangulation. This means that whenever the back is at an angle it is supported by the arms, or another part of the body. What is happening here is that the client's body and the plinth combine to transfer the weight down through the floor in an equilateral triangle. If the friction provided by the table against the floor and the client's body on to the table were not equal to the angle and force applied by the practitioner's body-weight and thrust, then the table would be pushed over.

Without this principle of triangulation the spine is unsupported and prone to injury.

Self Practise Exercise 18   One Triangle

Lean comfortably on a table with your back at a 45° angle and then remove
your arms, letting your back take the strain. Hold this until your back starts
to complain. Then replace your arms and slowly let them take your weight
once more, feeling the transference of strain down the vectors of the triangle
you have just created from your feet to your forearms and from your
forearms, through the plinth into the floor.

This exercise will allow you to focus all your awareness on the damage you may be doing
to yourself by not allowing your client to support your weight. In No Hands Massage,
then, this strain which can damage our backs is taken up by leaning on our arms and
thereby creating a triangulation of the vectors of force. To develop this leaning ability and
to counteract such damaging strain, carry out the following exercise:

Self Practise Exercise 19   Leaning

Standing beside your plinth, place your forearms on the surface without any
lean or pressure whatsoever. Experience the strain on your unsupported
back. Now relieve this strain by transferring your weight on to your
forearms. Experience the relief. Now further relieve your back by bending
your knees and dropping your hips lower down to the ground. Experience
the additional relief. Feel the vectors of force going into the table and down
to the floor through your feet.

This three-stage releasing exercise has saved the backs of many No Hands practitioners!
Once we have internalised the sensations we wish to achieve during bodywork, it becomes
possible to stay focused on self preservation during our massage sessions with even the
most demanding clients. By leaning on to our clients properly, we automatically employ
the principle of triangulation. By applying the principle of triangulation we automatically
lean properly on to our clients.

As an additional support to the principle of Triangulation, we can also employ the principle of 'Secret Levers'. It is possible during most strokes, to find additional support from the plinth. Using the table as a 'secret lever' in maintaining postural integrity is essential to the healthy practice of No Hands Massage. This means leaning hips, legs and upper body against the table in order to reduce any strain on the back. This is an essential component of triangulation. The belly, hips and legs of the practitioner, when braced against the sides and support structures of the massage plinth become valuable allies in the task of creating support for the spine during the massage. With these secret levers we are able to create 'mini-triangles' within the larger triangle shown above.

Self Practise Exercise 20   Multiple Triangles

Lean on to the far side of a plinth or table, creating a triangle with your arms and legs. This is your big triangle. Now bring up one of your legs and lean your knee against the plinth. Press your knee into the plinth. Feel the change in your back. Notice how it frees up your back to make movements that would otherwise have been a strain. Experiment. You have just created two triangles. Now place the foot of your upraised leg against your standing leg and let weight transfer into this as well. You have just created a third mini-triangle using the plinth and your standing leg as your 'secret levers'.

Many massage movements are not simply in one direction, but are circular and involve a complex set of muscle movements in the practitioner's own body. Secret levers can be employed to support all these movements in many different directions, even when they are not in line with the main thrust of the practitioner's stroke. Many strokes that I employ involve three or four additional triangles to reduce strain on my body.

Conclusion

When the principles of Verticality, Triangulation and Secret Levers are combined with the other postural principles, it is possible for the practitioner to apply powerful massage strokes without any damage to any body part. This is how we let all of our body-weight fall on to our clients and on to the floor. Any weight we hold back and keep to ourselves becomes a strain on our backs, and could be harmful, with repetition, over time.

Chapter 12   Postural Principle Six

Kneeling

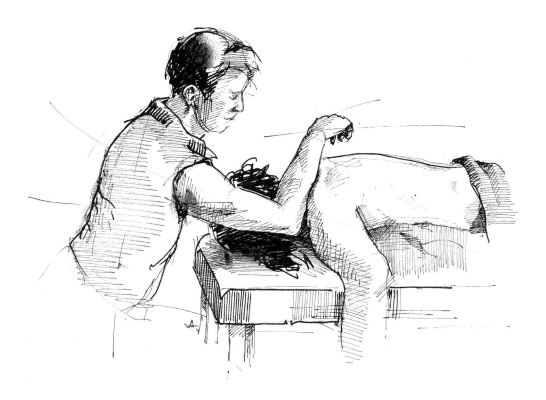

A revolutionary new posture

Kneeling makes it possible to apply powerful strokes with a vertical back with zero-strain to the practitioner. Unique to No Hands Massage, it is possible to now square the circle of effective massage with zero-strain to the practitioner. By kneeling, we can use our forearms to transfer the force transmitted by moving our hips and legs. 100% of the force for these strokes comes from the lower body, with the upper body in a relaxed and zero-strain position. The table has to be low for these kneeling techniques to succeed.

This is the most effective use of the principle of verticality, and although kneeling could be called a technique rather than a principle, it has so revolutionised the practice of massage therapists that it warrants a whole chapter on its proper postural execution.

Working upwards

Such vertical principles mean we can apply strong, powerful strokes by actually working *upwards*. This eradicates leaning and the need to concern ourselves with the distribution of upper body-weight *downwards*. Here, the back remains vertical throughout the stroke because the practitioner is kneeling. The stroke moves up from the knee and foot, with the pelvis providing the momentum and force for each stroke. The upward movement is provided by the upper arms, but because the arm is supported against the client's body there is no strain on the arm(1). In some ways the arm is simply trapped between the thrust of the practitioner's pelvis and the client's immovable body. As the practitioner's body moves closer to the client, the arm slides upwards and over the client's body. This means that the back remains vertical whilst strokes of considerable force are provided.

Powering 'up'

The power for this upward stroke comes entirely from the forward movement of the hips. This comes from a forward driving thrust from the trailing leg and a return to the beginning of each movement with a thrust from the leading leg.

Self Practise Exercise 21   Kneeling

Kneel with one knee back, and one foot forward on the floor, in what I call the 'proposal posture'. Place a cushion under the kneeling knee to protect it from any injury or soreness. Move your hips backwards and forwards keeping your back vertical. Enjoy the freedom and ease of these movements. THIS STROKE IS CONTRAINDICATED IF YOU EXPERIENCE ANY PAIN IN YOUR KNEE WHILST MAKING THE MOVEMENT. As you make the movement, lift your forearm vertically - this is how you are able to transfer the force of your hip movements on to the client's body.

Zero-strain

Kneeling vertical work can be done over most of the client's body, providing the table height is adjusted to the practitioner's body-size. This often means lowering the plinth to somewhere between the practitioner's knee and hip height. With the table thus adjusted, most of the client's muscle groups can be worked with force and pressure, whilst maintaining zero-strain on the practitioner's own body.

Work can be done on the spinal muscles, the arms, the gluteals, the adductor, hamstrings and abductors and the calf muscles and feet. In short, about 80% of the client's muscle bulk can be worked from kneeling. This is what is most revolutionary about No Hands Massage, namely the ability to work deeply and for a long time on most of the client's muscles, without any damage to the practitioner. The kneeling knee can be protected by placing a cushion on the floor or wearing trousers with knee padding. I always have a couple of pillows or cushions under the table, available to be quickly pulled out for such work.

These moments of verticality also provide the practitioner with much needed relief from the rigours of maintaining postural integrity whilst performing deep and effective massage movements using leaning. As these movements mainly involve dissipating strain from the back by supporting each 'lean' or 'falling over' and using the other six postural principles, this kneeling verticality provides a simple way in which to ensure that we are doing absolutely no damage to ourselves whilst working on clients.

Resting

Amongst the fell running fraternity in Hebden Bridge, we talk of "resting" whilst running downhill. This concept confused me at first as a novice runner. Yet once a certain level of fitness had been attained, I began to make sense of this paradoxical phrase. Clearly, to the observer, we are not resting but running downhill - in some cases quite fast. However by comparison with running up the craggy and boggy hillside, to the runner it is in reality a rest to come pelting downhill. Kneeling is similar - whilst clearly applying very powerful massage strokes, to the practitioner kneeling really does feel like a rest and a break from all the other postures.

Moving to a kneeling position also reminds us that *there are many different ways to apply the same stroke*. Changing our posture often is at the heart of all these principles. Such a principle is inherent in the principle of 'Flow' (see page 52).

Leaning and kneeling

Whilst a vertical spine is a zero-strain spine, our backs are able to take occasional strain - otherwise we would never move! By concentrating the bulk of our techniques on zero-strain approaches, we are free to experiment with some combinations of leaning and kneeling. Working upwards from the floor presents a whole new range of creative possibilities for the bodyworker.

Chapter 13   Postural Principle Seven

The Shire Horse

The shire horse of massage

In order to plough a heavily muddied field, our forebears used a shire horse, not a gazelle. How long would the gazelle have lasted? How much of the field would have been ploughed if a gazelle had been used rather than a shire horse? Yet this is exactly what I believe most bodyworkers are being trained to do, in using their thumbs and fingers and wrists to loosen large, tight muscles.

The secondary, tertiary and quarterly zones of the practitioner's body are the shire horses of bodywork (see Part 2). When combined with the whole body movements of the practitioner they are powerful tools for 'ploughing' the client's muscles.

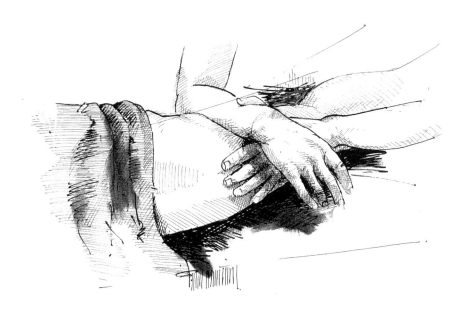

By 'plough' I mean the work of warming up, loosening, stretching, kneading and softening the soft tissue. Often, when this is done systemically throughout all the major muscle groups of the body, there is no need for further specific work.

The gazelle of massage

In contrast to the other zones, the primary zone (the palms, thumb and fingers) are the gazelles of massage. They have the sensitivity and finesse which enable us to palpate tiny knots and tensions in the body. Their precision enables us to make muscle-specific structural and energetic changes to the client's body. The palms can convey powerful warmth, healing and emotional reassurance as well as enable the practitioner to tune in to subtle shifts in the patterns of energy flowing within the client's body. Do not use a gazelle to plough a field! I am struck by the illogicality of using some of the smallest muscles in the practitioner's body (ie thumb and fingers) to massage the biggest muscles in the client's body (eg back and legs).

The shire horse equation

What this principle means in practice, is that we need to do our bodywork sums. To be octogenarian bodyworkers, we need to get these sums right. I believe that one important way of building a successful bodywork practice is by adhering to this principle, namely to ensure that:

> *The strength and weight of the practitioner's applied force must be greater than the tensile strength of the client's muscle being worked.*

where,

> S = Successful Practice
> P = Practitioner weight and strength
> C = Client's tensile muscle strength

this can be translated into the following equation :

$$S = P > C$$

In every session, and with every movement I make, I ask myself whether I have got this equation right. I know that if I have not then either I am damaging myself or my work is likely to be structurally ineffective. This is a usable equation that has proved of enormous value to many bodyworkers, and it represents the seventh principle in formulaic terms. When combined with the other principles, it can transform and lengthen a bodywork practice.

When working large, armoured muscles, our clients need us, in the main, to give them deep and repetitive work in order to loosen and stretch their ossified tissues. The question is: "Which muscles in my body am I pitting against which muscles in my client?". If working the massive hamstring muscles with the tiny digit muscles of the hand, what hope do we have of success? In military terms, this is the equivalent of taking on a Challenger tank with a pea-shooter.

Only by using our forearms and other parts of our body can we, in fact, apply large amounts of pressure without damaging ourselves. The beauty of the forearm is that it moulds so comfortably around many different parts of the body. The combination of the forearms, and the thoughtful positioning of our body-weight, will produce effortless working of tough muscle-groups in our client's body.

Vectoring

Once I started to think in terms of the amount of force and the direction of movement needed to *effortlessly* work the client's muscles, I began to think in terms of vectors of force. By this I mean mostly positioning my body behind the line of my movement. This sometimes means getting below my client and working upwards (see previous chapter).

The vectoring approach often means spending a little time shifting the body around, and trying out several different postures until you come up with a position that is comfortable for you. For myself, I believe that the preparation time taken before each stroke begins, communicates to my client how seriously I take the particular problems presented by them. It also conveys how committed I am to helping my client fulfil their structural contracts to release muscle tension.

Muscle surrender

Once I began to use the shire horse principle and its concomitant 'vectoring' something rather strange began to happen. As I worked out how to position my body and which part of my forearm I was going to use to transfer my weight on to my client's tight muscles, in the moment just before I leaned into the client, her muscles simply let go. At first I would carry on with the stroke, ignoring this vital piece of information. As it happened more often, I realised that my client's body was waving the white flag of surrender even before I started. It was as if the muscle was sensing the power and force being prepared to work on it and saying "Blimey, mate, I give in, honest!" without a struggle. As this has now become such a commonplace occurrence for me and my students, I offer it without explanation. It's a very Zen thing, though. As soon as I become 100% committed to applying every ounce of my body-weight in the service of facilitating release in my client's muscle, they release without any pressure whatsoever.

Chapter 14   A Summary Posture

The Dancing Bear

When all seven postural principles are followed, then often we find that the No Hands Practitioner is working in the 'Dancing Bear' stance. When we are breathing in our belly, and letting our weight drop down to the ground, and feeling each movement through our feet, leaning and falling over on to our client (or kneeling) and are operating support principles and shire horse principles, we begin to move rather like a bear. For this reason, if there is one postural image to hold in mind during bodywork, it is that of the "dancing bear".

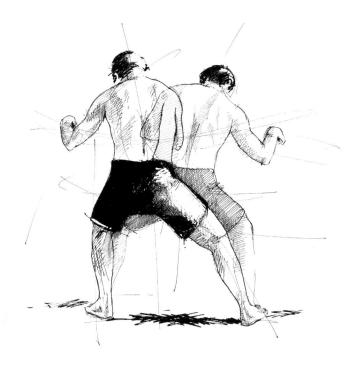

The most common features of this posture are: knees and elbows bent, head dropped forward, and the jaw is soft and loose. In this posture all the joints are 'open', that is, they are not locked rigid at full extension. This slight flexion of the joints means that there is maximum opportunity for flow of movement and energy in the bodyworker. When such flow and movement surrounds and touches the client's body, a quantum difference is introduced to the bodywork session.

1   Knees bent

No straight legs. In this way we transfer our body-weight down into the ground. Bending our knees, dropping down and engaging our strong leg muscles enables any tension and holding to be taken away from the back.

Rather than following ruler-drawn lines and images on a page, regarding our bodywork posture, I am advocating kinaesthetic and tactile *feeling* of our posture. This means paying attention to the internal sensations within our own body structure, as well as to the external sensations as we make contact with the table, the floor and the soft and hard tissues of our clients. It also means feeling and experiencing the transference of weight and energy into the ground. Stiffened joints actually block such awareness, as well as the flow of energy within our own bodies. As we lock the muscles surrounding a joint, we constrict nerve transmission, lymph and blood flow.

Self Practise Exercise 22   Locked Joints

Stand in the middle of the room with your eyes shut and your legs locked straight. Count to 10, and notice what you are aware of. Now slowly unlock both your knees, and notice the changes in your physiology. Has your breathing changed? Do you feel more energised when standing with knees bent or locked? Are you more or less aware of yourself and your body sensations now, or when locking your knee joints?

This principle of bent knees is central to No Hands Massage, and deserves regular practise.

Train Game

It is possible to practise this whilst standing in the tube or waiting for a bus. I play a game when travelling anywhere by train, which is to get ready for my station well before the train pulls in and feel the interplay between my different muscles as I try to keep my balance with knees bent and legs apart. If you find this easy, then you are obviously an advanced bodyworker and can now attempt the exercise on one leg with both eyes shut. Good luck!

2   Floppy wrists

Keeping the wrists floppy means literally letting them 'flap about'. This will ensure that the forearm musculature is kept soft, as it is these muscles which control wrist and hand rotation, flexion and extension. It will also enable the hands and wrists to be truly rested. More than this, it means the very same tightened muscles that may have contributed to wrist or finger pain are being massaged by the client's body. Concentrating on this floppy wrist principle also avoids the "clenched fist/ clenched jaw" attitudinal approach to relaxational massage which says to the client's body: *"You will relax!"*. If we stiffen or straighten our wrists when using our forearms, we tense the very part of the forearm that is used to apply the stroke, namely the soft front.

Any clenched fist tension reduces the malleability of the forearm and its wonderful ability to 'mould' around the client's body contours and protuberances. Such forearm tension also creates strain not only in the hand and wrist joints, but throughout the whole body. It is very hard to create tension in the hands and wrists without also tensing other areas of the body.

Self Practise Exercise 23   Systemic Tension

Try tensing now as you sit reading this: make a hard and tense fist and clench your jaw. Feel for any increase in tension elsewhere in your body. Depending on whether you are sitting, standing or lying down you may feel tension or even just the subtle echoes of tension in your shoulders, neck, lower back and hips. Even if you cannot feel any physical tension elsewhere in your body, simply notice the change in mood that such contractions induce.

It is possible to deliberately lock the wrist and fist to harden the forearm muscles to obtain a harder, firmer surface with which to massage, but this needs to be done with full awareness of the cost to ourselves.

Self Practise Exercise 24   Soft/Hard Forearms

Lean the soft front of your forearms against the edge of a table. Slowly clench and unclench your fists. Feel the changes in the surface of your forearms and the strain created in your wrist. Now do the same with the back of your forearms. The change is more subtle, but it is there nonetheless.

3   **Floppy head**

Another way to confront habits and patterns of tension in our own bodies during bodywork sessions, is to let the head roll a little whilst working. This physically loosens the muscles which 'hold our head up' in a certain way. Psychologically, it symbolises letting go of any rigidity of attitude we might have at this moment towards ourselves or our client. It also keeps us open to new and innovative ways in which to respond to the particular client's needs at this particular moment.

4   **Floppy jaw**

Keeping the jaw soft and loose is another of the secrets of keeping our whole body loose and relaxed whilst working. I do this by regularly rotating my jaw and stretching it during bodywork. This could be quite alarming to my client were they not lying face down or lying supine with their eyes shut! Often in my work with clients, I find that the key which unlocks tension anywhere in their body can be found in the jaw. By inviting my client - either verbally or non-verbally - to let go of their jaw, I find that hips and shoulders relax, and breathing often deepens. This is why it is important for me to regularly make movements which 'free the jaw', such as rotations and yawns. I believe the reason for the jaw being so central to our tension patterns is because so many of our childhood beliefs were based around what we thought we should or should not say.

The dancing bear posture

Now, before reading on, I invite you to do this final exercise, as a celebration of all the learning that you have absorbed so far. If you have done most of the exercises in this book, you will already have a kinaesthetic understanding of No Hands Massage, even before we look at seven massage strokes that utilise the principles of No Hands Massage.

Self Practise Exercise 25   The Dancing Bear

Stand in the middle of the room, let your knees and arms bend, drop your weight and flop your jaw, wrists and head. Breathe into this posture which encapsulates all the previous seven principles.

Chapter 15   The Philosophy of No Hands Massage

Introduction

Go deep, go slow

When applying large amounts of pressure to our client's muscles, it is imperative we do not trigger their "protection reflexes". This is when the 'fight or flight' response is activated. The response is a tightening and a hardening of the tissues and an increase in stress and tension to both the physiology and the psychology of our client. At this point we undo all the good 'opening' work we have achieved, and teach our client a lesson in not letting go and releasing. Rather like a trust exercise in which you are invited to fall back and trust your partner to catch you - if you are dropped and injured, it may take a while to trust that same person again. Even if a client consciously decides it's OK to have someone cause them pain, their unconscious, or 'somatic self', does not forgive so readily.

Any bodywork approach where pain and struggle and battle between client and practitioner are positively encouraged is the very antithesis of healing bodywork. Such an approach colludes with many of the negative belief patterns that people have thought the world over and throughout time in order to give themselves a hard time. Whilst the short term effects of such violent bodywork may be a release from pain, I believe the somatic message given to the client may be a very harmful reinforcing of such negative beliefs.

Changing change

When we inflict pain on our client, then we are in danger of colluding with negative thoughts. Likewise, when we invite comfortable and gentle release that is effortless, we empower our client to not only change, but to actually *change the way in which they make changes*.(1) The shire horse may be a powerful animal, but it is also a gentle giant of a beast.

The principle of going slowly if we wish our client to open up and let go of their tension, is really the fable of the tortoise and the hare writ large in the body. If we rush like a mad hare, busy with our dexterous techniques, thinking about "getting this muscle loose *whatever the cost*", then we often spend longer working on the client with less success.

Whenever I "go slow", take my time and communicate an unhurried dedication to my client, then I find that the whole atmosphere of my bodywork has an impact on muscle release.

Thus my attitudinal stance has an impact on my client's tissues. These attitudes of mine are transmitted unconsciously through the minutiae of my touch, the way I breathe and how I move my body. These messages are often received through my client's unconscious awareness. It does not matter whether either of us believe this happens - it happens anyway!

> *Yesterday I worked on a premier league footballer who was complaining of tightness and pain in his lower back and calves. As it was his first session I made a "let's see if this makes a difference" contract and gave him 30 minutes of No Hands Massage. As the minutes ticked by both he and I slowed down, and I dropped being the impressive bodyworker and showing off my techniques. Instead, I found myself slowing down and moving away from busy, deep structural work, and towards slow and gentle nurturance. I took his deepening breath and the* systemic softening and loosening of his muscles *as consent to this unexpected turn of events. By the end of thirty minutes he reported 'feeling a new man' and wanting to recommend me to the whole changing room. He felt no back or calf pain, and when asked what he found most effective said:*
>
> > *"The quiet and stillness of this lovely warm room and the space you gave for all of me to relax, not just my body."*

Ambient bodywork

I call this attitudinal awareness of which I have spoken 'ambient bodywork'. It consists of *the way* I give my bodywork, and this is driven by my beliefs about myself, others and life in general. These beliefs dictate how I give the bodywork I give. It is the impact I have on my clients *without even touching them*. Ambient bodywork also includes the better documented environmental components of bodywork such as: room temperature, aromatic smells, appropriate music, non verbal sounds such as sighs and overt breathing, lighting, decor, clean fluffy towels etc. Of all of these ambient techniques which bodyworkers employ, I believe that the most significant one is *the pace* of our work, and our own *attitude* to our clients.

Systemic massage

Very often, the structural complaints that people present in my massage room are the result of a systemic tension throughout their whole muscular system. If we use the analogy of clothing, the aches and pains they present actually show us where the fabric has torn, whereas the reason for tearing is that the material has shrunk. What my footballer was presenting was a tear in his clothes, and what I did was to give him a new, stretchy suit, rather than simply mend a single tear.

With No Hands Massage, systemic structural tightness can be achieved effectively and efficiently without any hurry. Once this systemic groundwork of loosening almost every muscle in the body is completed, the practitioner is free to attend to those areas of the client's body which have not rebalanced themselves naturally. This might mean focusing on specific structural or energetic blocks that both client and practitioner have identified. However, after such powerful systemic work, the client's own body often sorts itself out and restructures itself back into a more balanced postural configuration of muscle, tendon, ligament and bone.

Chapter 16   Seven Psychological Principles

No Hands Massage offers seven postural principles as solutions to some of the physical problems of bodywork. There is also a powerful psychological element to this system which deserves a mention here. There are at least seven psychological principles in action during every No Hands Massage session which explain why there is such a powerful psychological and emotional impact on clients from this bodywork form. Whilst each of these principles may be active in conventional massage, I believe that No Hands Massage intensifies their action.

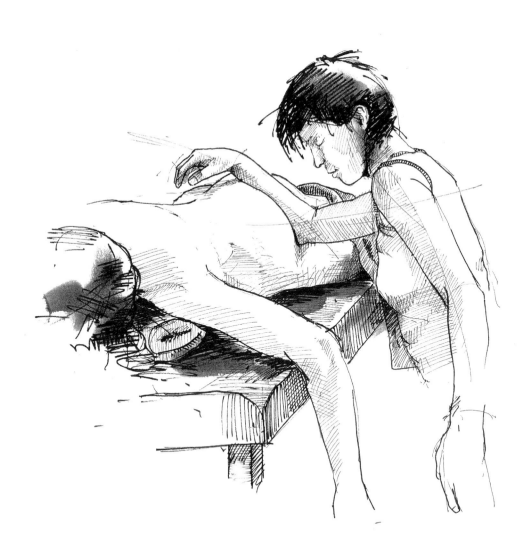

1   Attunement

No Hands Massage involves leaning our body-weight on to our client more than is normal in conventional bodywork. By leaning on our client, we not only avoid injury and strain, but we also create an environment conducive to the practitioner's attunement to the client's mental, physical and emotional state. This is achieved because when there is no pain and no strain for the practitioner, it becomes easier to 'tune in' to the client and sense the messages hidden within their body. We often feel these somatic messages from within our own body. There's nothing quite like leaning on someone to get a 'feel' for what's going on 'in there'.

Likewise, for the client, there's nothing quite like being leaned on to facilitate getting body-connected. The pressure of a practitioner's body-weight 'earths' the client and helps mind and body become reconnected. The more connected the client gets, the easier it is for them to ask for what is needed from the practitioner. This increased body-mind connection within the client also makes it easier for the practitioner to notice what is going on. It is as if the body's messages have been passed through an amplifier, by the increased pressure of No Hands Massage.

As we let our own weight fall on to our client, and use forearm techniques, we are also physically opening up our own chest area, the zone of our own heart Chakra. Because so many of the forearm movements in No Hands Massage involve the practitioner moving their arms laterally, opening up the chest, it mimics some of the most ancient healing exercises for "opening the heart" Chuen (1991, p. 68). In most movements you will find that the practitioner's chest is close to the client or in a very 'open' posture.

These movements, then, will energise the heart Chakra, the centre of compassion, and create a greater 'heart' connection between practitioner and client. Even on a purely physical level, the movements stimulate and exercise the chest muscles of the practitioner and physically open and free the structure of the whole thoracic region. As well as creating an 'open-hearted' posture, the physical opening of the thoracic region can also stimulate an open-hearted attitude through the link between body and mind.

Conclusion

The increased lean and physical proximity creates greater opportunities for the practitioner to attune to the client. The opening of the thoracic region, and repeated stimulation of the heart meridians, may also contribute to this attunement.

2   Intimacy

One of the reasons for attunement is that we are entering further into the client's personal 'space boundary' than is normal when using conventional techniques. The closer physical proximity produces an intensification of awareness of the client.

Conventional bodywork generally works one step in from the personal space boundary between two people, as defined by our western handshake. In conventional bodywork, the practitioner works at a level in which the client's space boundary and the practitioner's own space boundaries intermingle. Instead of touching the client's hand, the practitioner steps inside this boundary zone and touches the client's body. Such an intensified level of physical intimacy is one of the reasons why bodywork can be so fulfilling for the practitioner.

With No Hands Massage, bodywork takes place at least one joint (or forearm) even closer than conventional bodywork. Sometimes there is not even this space between practitioner and client. Such close intimacy is normally only achieved when holding or hugging another human being, in other words, when we are intimate.

The level of intimacy achieved through No Hands Massage can be positively exhilarating and/or threatening for the practitioner. Interestingly, on a conscious level, the client is often unaware of the proximity of the practitioner because great care is taken not to bump or touch the client with any part of the practitioner's body other than the intended 'contact' zone. This intimacy, then, requires an increased awareness and clarity regarding the personal boundaries between practitioner and client. I believe that the most tangible expressions of this client-practitioner boundary are threefold: our contact discipline, our draping, and our contracts and agreements with the client.

Contact

Because of the intimacy involved in No Hands Massage, practitioners need to develop an increased awareness of which parts of the body are in contact with the client. This means only the part of our body with which we have chosen to work is touching the client. Because the client is in a heightened sensory mode, even a small bump of the practitioner's hip or a brushing of clothing can become a major 'touch event'.

Draping and boundaries

I believe that the way we drape clients expresses how well we maintain clear boundaries in our relationships with them. Sloppy draping often expresses a lack of clarity regarding where work ends and personal life begins. Fussy draping often expresses a fear of contact and an over-rigidity of boundaries. Both are signs that personal work and supervision are needed in order to become comfortable with the complex job of being a massage therapist.

Contracts and boundaries

Another tangible aspect of dealing with this increased intimacy, is the need to become crystal clear regarding the scope and depth of the work between the practitioner and the client. For example, once a client has made a bodywork contract with the practitioner, without any further contract the practitioner has no right to pry further into the client's psychological state. The client may choose to give all sorts of information, but the practitioner should only be interested in this if it has an impact on the bodywork being given, and can be translated into actual bodywork movements. Anything else is 'therapeutic nosiness" and is better left to the psychotherapists, in my opinion.

Conclusion

The increased level of intimacy which is brought about by bodywork taking place one forearm closer to the client's skin, means that practitioners need to take great care about the boundaries of their relationship with a client. This can be done through being aware of contact, respectful draping and clear contracts.

3   Modelling 'Letting Go'

The probable aim of all practitioners and all clients is to 'let go' of tension. What is tension, other than an unnecessary and prolonged 'holding on' to our body-weight? In my experience 'holding on' is physical, mental and emotional. It is not for the bodyworker to define that this must be a 'physical only' release. It is the duty of the bodyworker to provide a secure environment in which the holding on can be released, in whatever way the client chooses.

This could mean letting go of physical tension in the shoulders, or it could mean letting go of the thought that 'people are out to get me' (often the belief accompanying raised shoulders), or it could mean a letting go of anger at a paranoia-inducing life history. It does not necessarily mean bashing cushions - the release of anger can often be witnessed as a sigh and a loosening of attachment to rage. Often, all three are released simultaneously and silently. It is for the client, and even the client's unconscious or 'somatic mind' to decide on the appropriate form of letting go.

The assured and sensitive release of the practitioner's weight on to the client's body has a powerful effect on the physical, mental and emotional state of the client. For the client, it becomes safe and appropriate to 'let go' of tensions on every level. When the practitioner displays enough body awareness and commitment to their art in order to transfer most of their body-weight on to the client, without causing any pain whatsoever, the client's body 'gets' that "*here is someone experienced and confident enough for me to let go*".

The practitioner, *by letting their own weight go* and leaning or falling over on to the client, models this 'letting go' to the client. As practitioners, we communicate on a subliminal level to our client that "letting go is OK". We convey physically that we have enough body awareness and confidence for them to safely hand over their body into our care and let go of their tensions, whether these are physical, mental or emotional. I have found that, as a client, when someone falls over on to my body it is hard to 'hold on'. The letting go of the practitioner's weight also expresses a very real mutuality in the client-practitioner relationship.

4 Mutuality

At each moment of bodywork, our client is actually supporting our unfolding just as much as we are supporting theirs. Falling over, then, is just one of the ways in which we let the bodywork we do reflect the essential inter-dependent nature of the client-practitioner relationship. This means that the No Hands Massage practitioner has a certain congruency about the way they work which "feels right" to the client.

Much talk is made of the imbalance of the power relationship between practitioner and client, with the practitioner seen as all-powerful. It is important that practitioners are aware of the potential for abuse in the relationship. The dependency of the client and the power of the practitioner is often seen in terms of the emotional and psychological needs of the client.

This mutual interdependence is, for me, one of the more important strands of the client-practitioner relationship. It is one of the reasons why I remind myself that our treatment contract is a two-way affair. If my client was not willing to play "client", then I would be unable to play "practitioner" in the game of life. This mutuality keeps me on an equal footing with my clients, and helps me avoid getting into either a "one up" or a "one down" position with clients(1).

5 Congruency and 'Walking the Talk'

By working on my clients without injuring myself, I am truly 'walking my talk'. This congruency increases the potency of my contact with clients. When my bodywork conveys 'be gentle with yourself' through touch and massage strokes, the effect of this is magnified because I am choosing to work in a way that does not injure me.

In this way, holistic principles of Mind, Body and Spirit are integrated into the very fibres of every No Hands movement. Holism is a concept that bodyworkers readily embrace in principle. How, then, is this principle actually incorporated into our bodywork movements? A holistic bodyworker should be recognised, not by their words, but by observing their movements during a session. No Hands Massage provides a tangible and disciplined way in which to bring such principles into the wordless language of the practitioner's own touch and movement. This is how our clients can actually 'feel' that we are truly walking the talk of self healing.

6   Commitment

There is little room for a tentative therapist in No Hands Massage. Any holding back of the practitioner's weight will increase tension and damage to the practitioner's body and convey tension to the client. To fall over expertly on to our client we need a psychological commitment to ourself, our work, our chosen bodywork *form* and our client. This commitment can be felt by the client through their tissues and nervous system during bodywork.

Receiving falling over bodywork, far from intimidating clients is mostly a profound relief for them. When was the last time, if ever, that they experienced touch from someone so committed and willing to put so much force, or weight, behind their touch? The answer is probably never. Even in the touch-rich period of our lives, namely when we were babies, such a ratio of touch pressure to client weight would not have existed. Such powerful, committed yet gentle, pain-free touch creates, I believe, a profound healing of any deficit of touch that we may have experienced at any time in our lives. Because the touch feels so big and powerful, we can easily regress into feeling 'little', and feed the parts of our past where we needed touch. All of this is happening, without client or practitioner necessarily intending it to happen. It is simply a pleasant and powerful experience.

It is also true that for some people, particularly with a history of abuse, this touch commitment *may* be a daunting challenge. Knowing, and sensing, how far and how much weight our clients are safe and happy with is part of the practical skill of No Hands Massage. Being aware of all the contraindications to this work is also part of the bodyworker's responsibility. This includes psychological and emotional contraindications as well as the purely physical ones. In general, the sensitive and gradual release of the practitioner's body-weight on to the client's body is experienced by clients as safe. For most it is an enormous relief, whatever their life history.

7   Hypnosis

Another reason for the potency of this "falling over massage", is that the continuous movement, the ebb and flow of weight and pressure has a hypnotic effect on the client. It creates a rhythm and dance all of its own which lulls the client into a state of release, in whatever form that release may take for the client at that moment. For some this may be sleep, for others a body that turns to jelly, and for others it may involve tears. Whatever is balancing for the client will surface through such gentle and hypnotic rocking.

I believe that such hypnotic bodywork lulls our internal 'guard' to sleep, and allows healing to sneak into the locked rooms and passageways of our psyche. I believe that this gentle rocking movement is a primal movement which releases the healer within each of us. Every time I lull my client into a hypnotic state through physical movement, I imagine their inner 'healer' escaping and getting to work on all their imbalances. Sometimes this is just a fantasy in my head which helps me to enjoy giving bodywork, and sometimes my client and I negotiate an explicit hypnotic contract for our bodywork, in which I will repeat certain agreed phrases during the session.

Either way, due to the increased whole body movements of the practitioner, No Hands Massage creates an increase in this hypnotic principle of massage.

自然

PART 3   SEVEN STROKES

The No Hands Massage training applies the four body zones available to the practitioner, with the seven surfaces of the forearm and the seven postural and psychological principles to almost every muscle in the body. This has resulted in over 60 different massage strokes, at least 40 of which are not documented elsewhere in bodywork literature, to my knowledge. This section shows seven of these strokes and how all the principles and theories of the preceding pages are actually put into action.

The name of each stroke is designed to be expressive of the movement as well as memorable or familiar in some way to practitioners. The seven massage strokes I have chosen replace some of the most damaging conventional effleurage, kneading and petrissage techniques. They are called:

1	**The Single Rolling Pin**
2	**The Hook**
3	**The Steamroller**
4	**The Arm Mangle**
5	**The Plane**
6	**The Stretchor**
7	**The Neck VW**

Chapter 17   The Single Rolling Pin

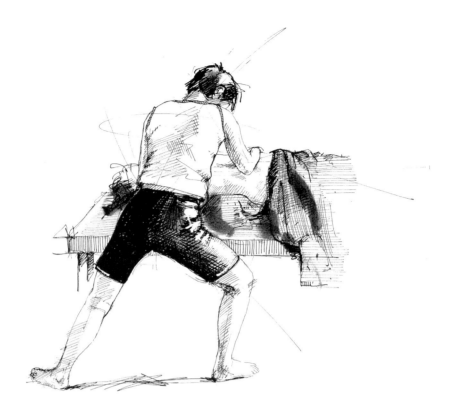

DESCRIPTION

This stroke applies the soft front of the forearm to the erector spinae muscles of the client's back. The soft front of the other forearm rests lightly on the client's shoulder or scapula during this movement. Because very little weight is transferred through the resting arm, the hand may be rested on the scapula.

Begin the stroke in the 'Dancing Bear' stance and then fall over, sliding down the back to the iliac crest, and return to the starting position by dropping your hips, bringing your spine to vertical, and using your legs to push yourself back to the client's shoulders, and the beginning of the next movement. The leg which is doing most of the work is the one nearest the client's feet.

Each stroke works down one side of the spine, without placing any direct pressure on the posterior spinous processes. The beginning of the movement is with your forearm contact starting around the client's T6. Your arm is at right angles to the spine, with your hand pointing slightly towards the client's head, and your elbow slightly towards their hips. The middle consists of sliding down the spinal muscles proximal to you, slowly bringing your hand out in an 'arc', away from your body, in order to ensure that contact with the client is through your soft front. The end of the movement is a circling over the iliac crest, where you draw the soft front towards you. Because the soft front of the forearm is used, there should be no 'bumping into' the client's ribs, spinous processes of the vertebrae or iliac crest with your ulna bone, and therefore no pain or discomfort for the client. Now, bring your forearm back, lightly pushing with your legs.

SAFETY AND CONTROL

If the pressure is too much for the client, or there is a sudden pain or a muscle spasm, then there is an instantaneous safety in immediately dropping your hips, thereby removing all weight going into your forearms. For you, the practitioner, the most damaging possibility is that you do not lean properly, hold your weight back and strain your own back. This is why the most relevant postural principle is 'Falling'.

POSTURAL PRINCIPLES

All the following postural principles are described in detail in Part 2 of this book.

Hara is utilised, primarily through breath. By letting the sound of your breath out through your mouth, you stay connected with your belly and how the movement originates from here. Throughout, the belly is central to all your movements, and in your leaning.

Feet The feet are used to experience and monitor the transference of weight forwards on to the forearms, on to the client, and sideways from one foot to the other as you travel down the client's back. All the force of your return is felt through the foot furthest from the client's head.

Flow This is a flowing stroke. There is a circular and hypnotic character to this movement, particularly if you also lean on your 'resting arm' as you transfer your body-weight back to the start position. This gives the whole movement a continuous feel for the client as there is always something going on.

Falling Your whole body-weight provides all the force necessary for this movement. Transferring your weight on to the client's body through your forearms supports your back. Whatever weight is not needed is transferred down to your feet. It is imperative that you do not strain your own back by 'holding back', and that you do not 'lift up' at the end of the movement, but rather drop your hips.

Support *Secret levers* are available from the side of the massage plinth throughout this movement, and *triangulation* is created between your feet, your shoulders and the floor via the client's body and the plinth. *Verticality* is employed at the end of the movement when your hips are dropped (bringing the spine erect without any strain to your back), and the knees bent. Weight is then transferred from the foot nearest to the client's hips, to the foot nearest the client's head, bringing your body back to the start position.

Kneeling This stroke is possible from the kneeling position, provided that the table is low enough. Care must be taken to 'drive' these kneeling movements from the hips, rather than the upper body, or arms.

Shire Horse The shire horse principle operates throughout this stroke. Your whole body-weight is targeted on the upper body muscles of the client. These erector spinae muscles need a lot of weight and a lot of work as they are continually being worked in response to different postures. They also have held minor and sometimes major misalignments for many years. For this reason, any effective work aimed at rebalancing these misalignments requires deep and repetitive pressure, something which would be permanently damaging to the fingers or wrists.

EXERCISE MOST RELEVANT FOR THIS MOVEMENT

Self Practise Exercise 16 Falling Over Bodywork

This technique uses the soft front (secondary zone soft anterior surface).

PHYSICAL EFFECTS

The falling over movement provides an effortless way with which to loosen and structurally open up the client's back, and it is often my first.

It is a deeply relaxing stroke and its effects are far superior to any effleurage that I know. The muscle fibres are worked smoothly and deeply, which both **warms and stretches the client's muscles**. This facilitates postural unlocking, unwinding and releasing. Getting to these deep tensions in such a pain free way gives this movement its potency. Normally such effective movements are accompanied by pain. Not so here. This movement allows the spine to realign itself naturally, providing the client has sought bodywork early enough. With a few sessions of this deep work, most clients can regain their postural balance and health without the need for other, more severe, interventions.

The depth of weight spread over the large soft surface of the forearm creates a passive stretch to the many different spinal muscles. As the muscles are being both stretched and 'worked' the fibres of the muscle are receiving a **Neuro-Muscular Technique**, in which the proprioceptive nerves to the belly of the muscle are being reprogrammed to 'rest' the muscle at a longer stretch. This has the effect of 'loosening' the vertebra and allowing for any re-alignment to take place naturally.

This stroke adequately **replaces conventional effleurage and petrissage** massage of the back. For this reason it can be returned to throughout the session, without any damage or discomfort to the practitioner. Each time the stroke is used, your work becomes deeper - both structurally and psychologically. Each time you use this stroke it also saves your back, as this is one of the most awkward twisting movements in the business.

PSYCHOLOGICAL EFFECTS

The Single Rolling Pin stroke provides a good opportunity to assess the client's psychological reactions to the unconventional contact of No Hands Massage.

Whilst all the psychological principles are present in all the strokes, the following principle is most in evidence here:

Commitment

Your commitment to this work is shown by the ease of your falling over, and the lack of any 'holding back'. The client will immediately become aware of any hesitation in transferring your weight on to the back.

Because of the amount of pressure being used, any mental 'holding on' becomes harder to sustain. It actually becomes easier for the client to let go of any negative beliefs they may have about bodywork, or themselves. The message is loud and clear "it's OK and safe to let go".

Through your awareness of your movements, and all the safety controls available, the client experiences the potency of this level of attunement. Not only are you aware of yourself, but you are also aware of the client's micro-responses. At the first sign of any discomfort, you can relate this awareness through a change in pressure which the client will immediately experience. The client realises they can be less 'watchful' as you are, in effect, saying to them "I will do the watching for you". A sigh often follows and a good chunk of the tension which the client arrived with has already dissipated in the first few minutes of the session.

This technique, then, is a good "Hello" stroke as well as being useful for deeper work if required. It can thus be used for nurturance or for the beginnings of deeper structural work. The amount of weight which can be applied through the stroke can provide a painlessly connecting and grounding effect for the client. Because of its flowing nature this stroke can also induce a deep mental relaxation and 'letting go' in the client, which I believe unlocks many of the tense spinal muscles responsible for minor misalignments and slight nerve impingement. In this way nurturance and structural techniques merge.

Chapter 18   The Hook

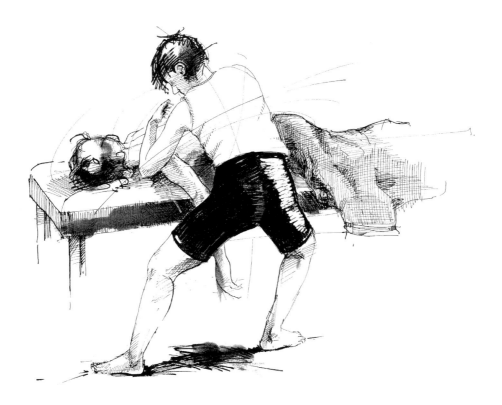

DESCRIPTION

All the power of this stroke comes from your own hip movements.

The stroke is achieved by placing your working arm on the erector spinae muscles of the client's mid-back (T8) and then moving your hips towards the client's shoulders, sliding your arm over the trapezius, leading with your elbow. It is completed by circling the shoulders and returning to the start position. To deepen the amount of stretch and postural realignment, you can 'hook on' to the client's whole shoulder girdle with both your lower and upper arm, forming an anterior V, and giving a powerful stretch by leaning your whole body-weight towards the client's feet, pushing with the leg you have nearest the client's head. Once this lean is completed, push with the foot you have nearest the client's feet in order to power a reversal of the movement and reach the start position once again.

SAFETY AND CONTROL

All weight and pressure can be instantly removed from the client by pushing into the ground with your feet and releasing all contact.

POSTURAL PRINCIPLES

All the following postural principles are described in detail in Part 2 of this book.

Hara This principle is active, primarily through your breath, as in the Single Rolling Pin. By letting the sound of your breath out through your mouth, you stay connected with your belly and how the movement originates from here. Throughout this stroke, the belly is central to all your movements and in your leaning.

Feet As in the Single Rolling Pin, the feet are used to experience and monitor the transference of weight forwards on to the forearms, on to the client, and sideways from one foot to the other as you circle the client's shoulder and then lean away. All the force of this lean is felt through your anterior V.

Flow This is a backwards and forwards semi-circular movement. There is also a pause as you lean and create a stretch to the shoulder girdle.

Falling Your whole body-weight provides all the force necessary for both phases of this movement. In the first phase, as in the Single Rolling Pin, your back is supported by transferring your weight on to the client's body through your forearms.

Support In the first phase of the movement, as in the Single Rolling Pin, secret levers, triangulation and verticality are all operative.

Kneeling This stroke is possible from kneeling. The kneeling position is restful for the practitioner, provided that the table is low enough. Care must be taken to 'drive' these kneeling movements from the hips, rather than the upper body or arms.

Shire Horse This principle operates throughout the stroke. You are using your upper body-weight to work the shoulder girdle muscles. Your arm is used in a 'lock' position, so there is some tension from such a static hold, but this requires much less effort than working the client's shoulder girdle with your hands.

EXERCISE MOST RELEVANT FOR THIS MOVEMENT

Self Practise Exercise 6 The V

ZONES/PARTS OF BODY USED

Secondary and Tertiary

PHYSICAL EFFECTS

This is a major upper body massage technique. Hardly any muscle from the diaphragm
up is untouched. Employing your whole body-weight to pull the shoulder away from the
head effectively works and loosens all the muscles responsible for neck and head tension, as
well as any restriction of breathing.

Most conventional techniques for this shoulder girdle, trapezius, rhomboid, pectoral
complex rely heavily on the fingers and thumbs, and for this reason, use of the Hook will
add years to your clinical practice.

PSYCHOLOGICAL EFFECTS

Because of the shire horse principle, here seen at its most potent, resistance is futile and
muscle surrender very common (see page 72, para 1). Letting your shoulder position be
readjusted often reflects a reappraisal of your need to 'shield' yourself from the world. The
shoulder girdle is used to lift the 'shield' of your scapula to ward off blows. Very often this
powerful work is accompanied by a deep sigh as the client, either consciously or
unconsciously, 'gets' the safety of this massage moment.

Such a realisation, that in the 'now' there is very rarely anything stressful going on, is a
major somatic therapeutic achievement. In the 'now' of this massage moment, what
possible reason could there be for shielding? You invite your client to give their 'inner
warrior' time off from the arduous task of protecting the self from invasion.

Whilst all the psychological principles are present in all the strokes, the following principle is most in evidence here:

Attunement

The client will feel the level of your awareness of all their tensions and holding patterns. The more attunement you show to the client's physical holding patterns, the more they will feel safe to let go on every level. It is very hard to let go of shoulder protection on a purely physical level.

Chapter 19   The Steamroller

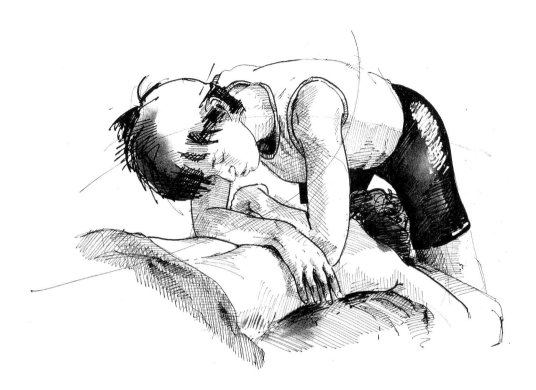

DESCRIPTION

This stroke uses both forearms to work the erector spinae muscles on both sides of the spine simultaneously. Care must be taken when at full extension not to bump the client's head with your pubic bone. This is one of those strokes which looks very intimate, yet to the receiver there is often no awareness that the practitioner is even on the table.

The Steamroller stroke is achieved by placing both of your 'soft fronts' on the spinal muscles, either side of the spine, level with T4/5. By pushing with your legs and keeping your back straight, you can slide down the client's back, distributing your body-weight between your knees and your forearms. When you reach the sacrum, circle over the iliac crest, and down to the gluteal muscles by dropping your chest lower to the client's body. Then, pulling from your hips, drag your arms back along the client's sides, and your forearms back over the ribs, pushing up from your hips and arms to avoid any back strain to yourself.

SAFETY AND CONTROL

All weight and pressure can be instantly removed from the client by dropping your elbows on to the table. Finer adjustments can be made by sinking more or less weight into your hips and knees and pushing your arms forward. When you are right above your forearms the pressure is maximal. This same place on the client's back can now be worked lightly, by leaning your weight into your hips and stretching your arms forward.

POSTURAL PRINCIPLES

All the following postural principles are described in detail in Part 2 of this book.

Hara This principle is active, as you are carrying your belly over the client's body (without touching). Your awareness of this 'Hara movement' is at the heart of the sensitivity and awareness that you can bring to the transference of weight from your knees to your forearms.

Feet In this case the 'feet' principle is experienced through the knees and any portion of your lower leg that is in contact with the table or floor. Paying attention to the amount of weight on your knees will increase your awareness of the part your hips are playing in the movement.

Flow This principle is evident in both the flowing way in which you can climb on to and off the table, and in the manner in which you make the transition from going forwards into going backwards. The arms flow down the back and then circle over the hips and are pulled back by your whole body movement. This makes it a very flowing movement, as well as a structurally powerful one.

Falling Your whole body is committed to this movement, and this is the very epitome of the principle of "falling over on to your client". Whilst the receiver may indeed experience the effect of this massage stroke as similar to being pleasantly 'steamrollered', the practitioner experiences it being more akin to 'skiing down the slope' of the client's back. Your forearms support your back throughout the movement. In order that you do not injure your back as you return to the start position, drag your upper body-weight back by leading the return from your hips. As this involves lowering your hips closer to the table, you must only do this if you have plenty of clearance between your hips. *This stroke must not be attempted unless all contact between your hips and the client's head can be avoided.*

Support In this stroke, you are totally supported by the table and the client's back. Triangulation is also operative, as can be seen by drawing a line between your knees, your shoulders and your forearms.

Kneeling This stroke is made from a kneeling position, and the soft surface of the tabletop should give enough protection for most practitioners' knees. It is a double kneeling position as opposed to a single kneeling position, which is fine as there is no need for any sideways movement by the practitioner.

Shire Horse This principle operates throughout the movement. By driving the movements of this stroke from your legs and hips, and using the whole of your bodyweight to apply pressure you are ensuring that the shire horse equation is adhered to, namely that $S=P>C$.

EXERCISE MOST RELEVANT FOR THIS MOVEMENT

Self Practise Exercise 14 Crawling Bodywork

ZONES/PARTS OF BODY USED

Secondary Zone: The 'Soft Pads' of the forearm are used because without them this amount of weight would hurt and even damage the client.
Tertiary Zone: During the 'drag back' the upper arm massages the sides of the client's back.

PHYSICAL EFFECTS

This is a major upper body massage technique. It provides a passive stretch combined with working over the muscles with considerable force if necessary. The stroke produces a Neuro-Muscular effect, in which the muscle is stretched and worked simultaneously. This tricks the brain into programming itself to lengthen the muscle.

No pressure is applied to the posterior processes of the spine itself, the soft pads of the forearms are tracking down two inches to each side of the spine, working the erector spinae. Because of the power of this massage stroke, the client experiences it as an effective 'ironing out' of most muscle tension and of the many small muscle 'knots' in the back.

This deep stroke clearly lengthens and relaxes many postural muscles with all the benefits that this brings to the nervous system. It replaces most effleurage and petrissage techniques of the hands. By relaxing and straightening the spine, many of the minute restrictions to both nerve and lymph flow are removed, thereby increasing overall balance and self-healing.

This is also a 'touch rich' stroke, as so much of the practitioner's arms (secondary and tertiary zones) are used during the movement. This is especially true during the 'drag back'. Thus the client receives a massive amount of sensory nerve stimulation with all the concomitant physiological and psychological implications.

For the practitioner, the movement provides a nice stretch, particularly to the lumbar and thoracic regions. The release of upper body-weight on to the client can also produce a realignment of many bones in the practitioner's own spine, thereby straightening out 'Janet' as well as 'John'.

PSYCHOLOGICAL EFFECTS

Whilst all the psychological principles are present in all the strokes, the following principle is most in evidence here:

Commitment

Whether or not the client consciously realises that your whole body-weight is committed to the movement, their 'somatic mind' will be registering the power and fluency of such competent body movements. The sheer depth and weight contained within this stroke makes 'letting go' much easier and more comfortable than 'holding on'. This letting go is as much a psychological event as a purely physical one.

Chapter 20   The Arm Mangle

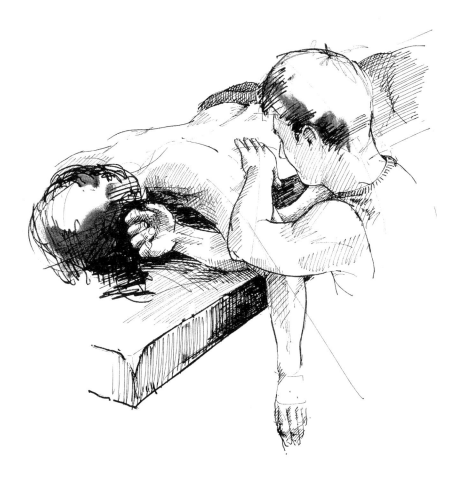

Description

The arm mangle uses the soft front of your forearm, combined with the soft tissue of your upper arm (relaxed biceps) to make a V or 'crook' in which you place the client's upper arm. By placing the soft front of your other arm over the client's arm you create a virtual 360-degree coverage or 'mangle' of the client's arm. Ensuring that you have previously covered both the client's arm and your own arms with sufficient oil, slide down the arm, gently squeezing the soft tissues in the client's arm. End the stroke by massaging the palm of the client's hand, creating a gentle traction to the shoulder joint. By resting your lower arm on your knee, you save yourself any strain whatsoever in this movement.

SAFETY AND CONTROL

The amount of pressure on the client's arm is controlled by the amount of downward pressure you apply by 'leaning into' your upper arm.

POSTURAL PRINCIPLES

All the following postural principles are described in detail in Part 2 of this book.

Hara This principle is active, primarily through your breathing and your kinaesthetic connection with your own movements and the client's somatic responses.

Feet In this case the 'feet' principle is experienced through one knee (the 'down' leg) and one foot (the 'up' leg). The knee of your 'up' leg carries all the pressure of the stroke when massaging the lower arm.

Flow This principle is evident in the way in which the stroke flows down the client's arm.

Falling Your whole body is committed to this stroke. Your arms form a grip which enables you to hold on to the client, the more you lean, the more you hold on.

Support There are many hidden supports in this stroke. The table forms a useful 'secret lever' against which you can lean your shoulder at the beginning of the stroke. The client's arm is your major support during the stroke. When you are leaning, and when you are pressing down on to the client's forearm, your own knee provides an important support.

Kneeling This whole stroke is designed to be done from kneeling, thereby making zero-strain to your back possible.

Shire Horse This principle operates because you are using the whole of your upper body-weight to apply pressure. The use of your whole body-weight to apply pressure at the beginning and traction at the end of the movement, creates an environment in which it is easy for the client to 'let go'.

EXERCISE MOST RELEVANT FOR THIS MOVEMENT

Self Practice Exercise 21   Kneeling

ZONES/PARTS OF BODY USED

Secondary Zone: The 'Soft Pads' of the forearm.
Tertiary Zone: The soft tissue of the upper arm.

PHYSICAL EFFECTS

This stroke provides a powerful mobilisation of the whole shoulder-neck complex. By leaning towards the client's head at the beginning of the stroke, the shoulder is pushed towards the client's head. By leaning your whole body-weight away from the client's head at the end of the stroke, whilst still holding their hand in a 'mangle', you create a powerful traction to the whole limb.

The stroke adequately replaces all effleurage strokes of the arm and hand, providing an efficient 360-degree coverage. When pressing or massaging over certain parts of the arm, leaning as you do so, you also replace petrissage and compression strokes.

PSYCHOLOGICAL EFFECTS

Whilst all the psychological principles are present in all the strokes, the following principle is most in evidence here:

Intimacy

This principle predominates as there is a certain amount of intimacy in having your upper arm hooked under the client's upper arm. Your shoulder comes very close to the client's shoulder. This intimacy if often experienced by the client as structurally powerful and nurturing.

Chapter 21   The Plane

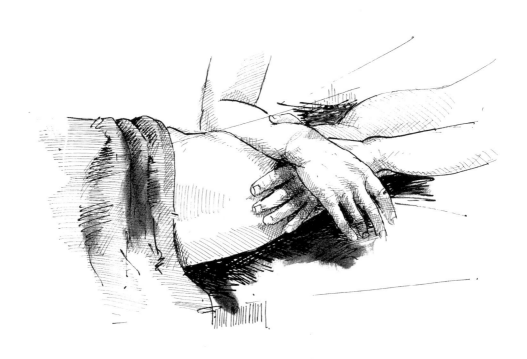

This stroke can be made standing, or kneeling, depending on preference and table height. It massages the posterior, lateral and medial muscles of the upper leg, as well as the calf muscles.

The word 'Plane' refers to the carpentry tool which scoops layers off planks of wood. The stroke can be used in two different ways, one encompassing the lower leg and the other encompassing the upper leg.

The stroke can produce a thorough working of the major leg muscles. By leaning your whole body-weight into the stroke, you produce a very deep pain-free massage of the hamstring, adductor, abductor, gastrocnemius and soleus muscles of the leg.

Your side hand acts as a 'guide' for this stroke, and does not have any real pressure transferred into it. At most, it provides a low-strain effleurage to the client's tissues. It also contributes greatly to the overall security and completeness of the stroke. By acting as 'guide' along the lateral surface of the client's leg, it gives stability to the action. The force of the stroke is transmitted through the soft front of your forearm. The beauty of this stroke is that with the sensitive variation of force and pressure you can work the client's leg muscles deeply and effectively. By altering the angle of your forearm, you can work both the adductors and the abductors very deeply.

As in the Single Rolling Pin, you transfer your weight on to the client's body, as you fall over. Be very careful to always have support for your back whenever you lean forwards. When standing, your own forward leg and the client's leg provide support. When kneeling, support for your back is provided by your forearm, the client's leg and your own knee and foot.

SAFETY AND CONTROL

You control the amount of pressure through the amount of your lean. When doing this stroke standing, you can simply fall off the client on to the plinth or floor in an emergency. If you need to reduce or adjust the amount of weight you are transferring on to the client's leg, do this by transferring more or less weight into your leg.

POSTURAL PRINCIPLES

All the following postural principles are described in detail in Part 2 of this book.

Hara The main movement is not in the arms at all. The main movement occurs in your belly, driven by your legs and hips - which gives power to this deep and effective massage stroke.

Feet When standing, your feet act as a pivot for your body to lean on to the client. By monitoring and paying close attention to the sensations in the soles of your feet, you remain aware of the continual movement and flow of the stroke.

Flow This stroke has a rhythmic 'to and fro' feel to it. It powerfully massages some of the biggest muscles in the body. It is possible to effortlessly repeat the stroke for as long as necessary; the stroke falls into the category of 'zero-strain' when done from the kneeling position.

Falling This principle is operative. The whole force of the 'Plane' is provided by the controlled fall on to the client's leg.

Support When standing, the table becomes a useful 'secret lever' against which you can lean your legs during the stroke. Triangulation is similar to the Single Rolling Pin, in that a triangle is formed between your shoulders, your feet and the client's body. The most supportive part of this stroke is provided either by your own forward leg or by the client's legs. By holding your weight back you risk serious damage to your own back.

Kneeling When done from a kneeling position, the 'Plane' becomes a 'zero-strain' technique. Your kneeling leg acts as a pivot as you let your body-weight fall forwards on to the client, and your 'up' leg (the one where your foot is on the floor and your knee bent) drives the return of your body back to the beginning of the stroke.

Shire Horse This principle is operational in that you are working the large leg muscles of the client with your whole body-weight. As it is the leg muscles which support the whole body-weight, this seems appropriate and fits within the shire horse equation of S=P>C. (see page 71).

EXERCISE MOST RELEVANT FOR THIS MOVEMENT

Self Practice Exercise 16 Falling Over Bodywork

ZONES/PARTS OF BODY USED

Primary Zone: The palm of the hand (lightly)
Secondary Zone: The 'Soft Pads' of the forearm.

PHYSICAL EFFECTS

This stroke effectively replaces many tiring palmar effleurage techniques, as well as conventional kneading techniques. In addition to saving the hands, this technique also avoids any twisting in your back, as you are facing in the direction of the stroke.

The stroke can be very light or very deep. The Plane can be used as effectively for nurturing touch as for a deep 'mulching' of the muscles.

All the tissues of the leg will be well worked after only a few of these strokes, and the power of the strokes means that the client feels that their whole body is being pushed and pulled up and down the table. Actual movement over the table is almost non-existent. This is a very time-efficient stroke, as a great deal of massage work is achieved in a very short space of time, and means that the practitioner can work in an unhurried way.

PSYCHOLOGICAL EFFECTS

Whilst all the psychological principles are present in all the strokes, the following principle is most in evidence here:

Mutuality

The easy transfer of your weight on to the client's legs communicates the interdependence of the client-practitioner relationship. The client's tense muscles have to 'yield' for you to be effective.

The psychological impact of this stroke is often one of relief. Very often, the recipient can experience tension in the legs as pain or ticklishness. With such a soft wide surface to transfer pressure on to, there can be deep structural release without any pain or tension. The application of safe draping techniques enables the client to relax into deep work, even on the inner thigh. Safety and boundaries are thus communicated on both a psychological and a physical level.

Chapter 22   The Stretchor

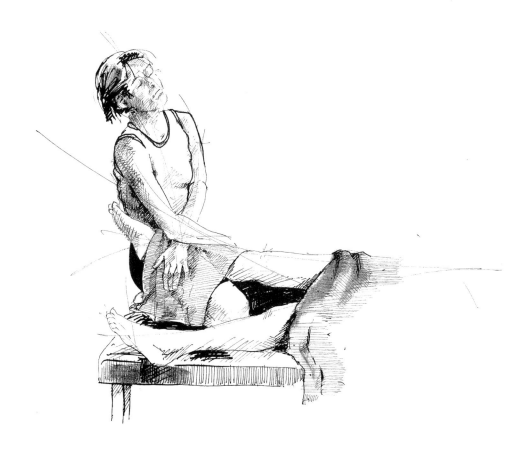

DESCRIPTION

In 'The Stretchor', a firm pressure is applied through your forearms on to the client's leg, which is hooked over your own hip. As you lean your body-weight backwards you pull your client towards you creating whole body traction without any strain to your hands.

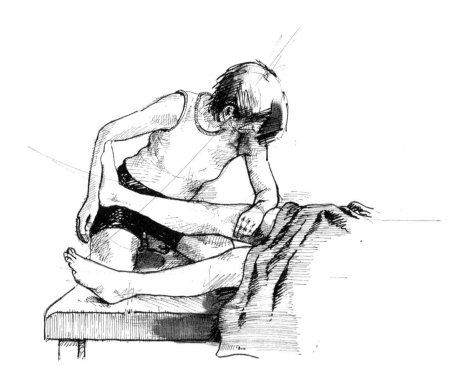

A lovely balancing move can be added in between each stretch by leaning forward and placing your forearms on the sole of the client's foot. This creates a compression of the hip and spinal joints.

SAFETY AND CONTROL

Release the client's leg.

POSTURAL PRINCIPLES

Hara This principle is active as the Hara acts like a magnet, dragging your client's weight and energy with each movement you make.

Feet This is experienced through your contact with the table and the floor, whatever position you find that is comfortable for you.

Flow This can be a powerful rocking movement.

Falling Whether falling backwards or forwards this principle is active.

Support Totally supported by the table.

Kneeling This is like feet, it is dependent on your final posture.

Shire Horse Not only do you have your whole body-weight to apply traction and compression, but also your active upper body rocking. This gives you quite an edge over your client's passive body-weight.

EXERCISE MOST RELEVANT FOR THIS MOVEMENT

Self Practise Exercise 13 The Flow of Stillness

ZONES/PARTS OF BODY USED

Secondary & Quarterly

PHYSICAL EFFECTS

Giving traction and compression to the client is a high stress technique for bodyworkers. Not any more.

For the client the ebbing and flowing of compression and traction creates an environment conducive to connection when the strokes are done slowly enough. This hypnotic stroke facilitates many physical and psychological releases.

PSYCHOLOGICAL EFFECTS

Whilst all the psychological principles are present in all the strokes, the following principle is most in evidence here:

Hypnosis

This stroke can have a powerful hypnotic effect on the client. The effortless and rhythmic movement of the whole of the client's body is conducive to inviting the client into a deeply receptive trance-state.

Chapter 23   The Neck VW

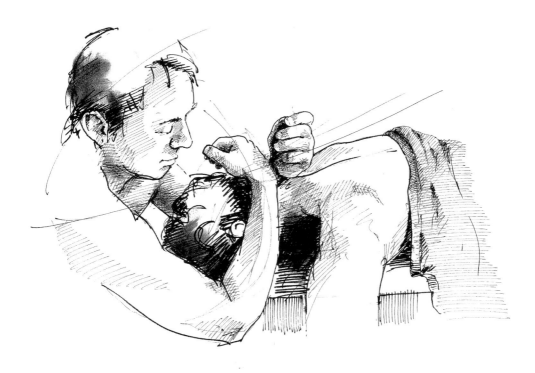

DESCRIPTION

This stroke uses the small hooks or epicondyles at the distal end of the lower arm (radius and ulna). These are the two bumps at the base of your wrist joint, one below the thumb, one below the little finger. They can be felt by running one hand down your lower arm just before you reach the wrist.

From a sitting or kneeling position, place your elbows on to the plinth and place these 'hooks' gently into the base of the client's skull. By leaning backwards, you can provide a powerful traction to the client's neck and spine.

All weight and pressure can be instantly removed from the client by leaning forward.

POSTURAL PRINCIPLES

Hara The 'lean-back' which provides a whole body stretch is achieved by focusing on your Hara. Sometimes this is more of an energetic pull than a physical one.

Feet Through your contact with the ground, you monitor your weight transference and your 'form'.

Flow This stroke has a more subtle flow to it than a large effleurage stroke. Working the top of the neck is most effective when done gently and rhythmically, like waves breaking down the cliff face.

Falling This stroke involves 'falling off' the client, rather than a falling over.

Support The plinth top provides upper body support, because your elbows can rest there. The plinth legs provide leverage for your hips, belly and legs. Verticality is operative.

Kneeling This is a kneeling stroke, and movement is powered from below the hips.

Shire Horse Your whole body-weight is used to stretch the whole of the client's body.

EXERCISE MOST RELEVANT FOR THIS MOVEMENT

Self Practise Exercise 13 The Flow of Stillness

ZONES/PARTS OF THE BODY USED

Secondary Zone: The small hooks of the lower arm (styloid processes at the distal end of the radius and ulna).

Physical Effects

This stroke creates traction to the whole upper body as the weight of the client's hips acts as the anchor on the table. The client should experience no pain or discomfort. As most conventional tractions are applied with the practitioner's fingers, this forearm technique eliminates any possibility of digital damage.

Psychological Effects

Whilst all the psychological principles are present in all the strokes, the following principle is most in evidence here:

Attunement

This principle is active in that the way you apply traction communicates your level of awareness and attunement. As the client experiences your connection with your own body movements, so it comes clear how attuned you are to their subtle tissue responses. In this respect, 'modelling' is also an active psychological principle.

This stroke can create a deeper connection between mind and body, as it works on the occipital ridge - often regarded as the body's physical representation of the gateway between the two.

自然

PART 4 CLINICAL CONSIDERATIONS AND
THE BENEFITS OF
NO HANDS MASSAGE

Chapter 24   Clinical Considerations and Contraindications

No Hands Massage is an advanced bodywork technology that assumes knowledge of the main contraindications to bodywork. What follows are some additional clinical considerations which are unique to No Hands Massage.

1   Greater proximity to client

Greater physical proximity between client and practitioner can create a few problems for client and bodyworker alike.

Using forearm massage generally brings the practitioner's body approximately 18 inches closer to the client. Conventional massage does not normally intrude into this space. However, it should be noted that even in conventional massage applications these boundaries are often dissolved by the time a face massage is given.

Clients who struggle with the intimacy of conventional (arms-length) strokes are contraindicated for No Hands Massage, due to the possibility of psychological 'overwhelm' or claustrophobia that this could cause them. No Hands Massage in this situation would be an intrusion and possibly a violation.

What is important is that the practitioner enters into the client's personal space gently and by degrees, always paying attention to the subtle holdings and tightenings which occur when there is anxious discomfort or a sense of invasion in the client. Unless a bodyworker has been trained to spot these subtle tightenings, they should not attempt No Hands Massage. In addition, if the bodyworker finds this proximity uncomfortable for themselves, even after several No Hands bodywork sessions, it is important they stop.

Respecting one's own comfort/discomfort zones is as important as respecting them in the client. If a practitioner wishes to work with the intimate power of No Hands Massage then they may need to seek out psychotherapy or counselling to identify and resolve the cause of any difficulties. Such difficulties may likewise be resolved through receiving No Hands Massage regularly from a practitioner skilled at noticing anxieties in the tissues of the body, and who is able to work safely and contractually at the edge of the anxiety.

2 Hygiene

Personal hygiene standards have to be maintained even more strictly with these close proximity techniques than in conventional 'arms length' massage. Smelly arm-pits, halitosis, smoky breath, greasy hair and dirty clothes become even more offensive in No Hands Massage, due to the closer proximity of the practitioner.

3 Body contact

No Hands techniques encompass all four zones of the body. It is essential that only the part of the body being used for the stroke is in contact with the client. Because of whole body use and greater proximity to the client, the practitioner has to be even more adroit at avoiding contact with other parts of the client's body. For female practitioners, bumping breasts against the client is an obvious example. Extreme care must be taken to maintain an air of professionalism throughout these applications and NO OTHER BODY CONTACT is advisable, apart from that which is intended.

> ### Sensory and Motor 'modes'
>
> *When I am receiving bodywork, I am primarily in a sensory-nerve receptive state. My sensory nerves are flooding my brain with a rich variety of stimuli as a result of the bodywork. When I am giving bodywork, however, I am primarily in a motor-nerve receptive state. I am primarily monitoring my* movements *during bodywork, through the feedback I am getting from my muscle nerve receptors.*
>
> *When I accidentally 'bump' my client with a part of my body, this is a small event in my 'motor-nerve' perception. For my client, however, who is in a heightened sensory receptive state, it is a major sensory 'touch event' and could be interpreted by them in many different ways. Part of keeping clear boundaries with clients is keeping my touch within the confines of our agreed therapeutic contract.*

4   Psychological contraindication

Clients who show signs of struggling with the client-practitioner boundaries, are contraindicated for this more intimate style of bodywork. The signs for this psychological contraindication are numerous. I am thinking here of the client who lingers at the end of the session, despite clear indications that it has ended. Some clients display this boundary confusion by repeatedly inviting their bodyworker out to social engagements. Other clients ask lots of personal questions. Some arrive late. Others arrive early. Some don't pay up, some pay three months in advance. Some clients keep changing their appointments and others make frequent and unnecessary phone calls. All of these may be signs of a possible struggle with boundaries.

These clients may actually find this closer proximity distressing or confusing. Some, for example, may well misinterpret this closer proximity as an invitation for sexual intimacy. No Hands techniques need to be monitored very carefully for any such negative effect they may be having on a client, or on the client-practitioner relationship.

5   Changes

If a client is used to conventional massage applications it can be a surprise and even a shock to have a practitioner leaning over and using their body in a creative way. It may be necessary to prepare the client by mentioning that sometimes the forearm will be used during the massage and that they are to give immediate feedback of any discomfort with this.

Remember, however, that the practitioner's interest and excitement with No Hands Massage may also be the very reason why this client has chosen them, because of the practitioner's ongoing commitment to their own professional development. The client may be there *because* the practitioner has built up a reputation for being innovative and creative in their massage applications!

Sometimes, particularly with the anxious client, it may be better to gently and gradually introduce the new techniques without any build up. I have done an 80% No Hands Massage on a client who had only previously had conventional techniques, without her noticing I wasn't using my hands. These techniques look more different than they feel. Because the practitioner is moving very differently, it doesn't follow that the client will notice this. They will only feel a depth and an awareness to the work. At the end of the day, only the practitioner will know what is going to be the most effective and appropriate way to introduce these new techniques to their clients.

It is not necessary, in my opinion, to ask for the client's consent for the choice of every technique used. Providing the work produces the outcome the client seeks, and causes no pain, I believe the client consents to the bodywork by staying on the table and *physically consenting* to the work. All my clients are tutored in their responsibility to communicate anything that is uncomfortable for them.

6   Depletion

There is no doubt that whilst this approach protects the practitioner's back, wrists and fingers, it also involves greater use of the whole body and, therefore, requires a greater input of energy. This is true of the muscles in the lower half of the body, especially the thigh muscles. On the whole, the increased activity actually creates energy, as much tiredness results from blocked and congested energy. Whenever I feel tired I put even more attention into the form, discipline and flow of my movements, and I find it mobilises my energy.

However, if the practitioner is in a truly depleted state, no amount of healing movements can replace the simple and basic human need for rest; the vigorous new strokes and accompanying movement *can* deplete further. If the practitioner finds themself working when depleted, then it is probably a good idea to raise the table and revert to less energising conventional techniques.   If the practitioner is so depleted, however, it may be time to question massaging at all. If the practitioner is not looking after themself then they are giving a mixed message to their client: on the one hand they are saying "Look after yourself" and on the other, they are saying "Look, I don't!".

Nowadays, if I have to cancel a client due to my own deplection, I am consicous if what good modelling I am providing: this models that it is 'OK' for us to place our own needs above the demands of others.

7   Forearm insensitivity

Initially, the practitioner may find it hard to "feel" what is going on in their client's body, especially if they have not used their forearm much before during massage. There are fewer sensory nerves in the whole of the forearm than in the palm of the hand. This could mean that in the early days if the practitioner is not careful, they may miss the client's physiological responses to the pressure being used.

Whenever doing deep work in the early stages, I train my students to keep one hand flat, acting as a 'sensor'. Using the hand as a sensor involves a process of retraining the brain to pay more attention to different sensations and cues. After a couple of years practitioners find that they are picking up as much (if not more) from their clients, through their whole body awareness, much like some deaf people 'hear' with their whole body.

8   Full body-weight

As most movements involve the use of the practitioner's whole body-weight, there is an increased possibility of damage to the client's soft tissues. This is why for every movement taught on the No Hands training, we also teach a 'safety'. 'Safeties' involves a support or an escape route which the practitioner can take in order to immediately remove all their weight from the client's body *at the first sign of discomfort.*

However, if full body awareness is practised and the soft proximal surface of the anterior forearm is used long enough to develop full sensory awareness of the client, then this safety 'escape route' for each stroke should not be needed. Such full body awareness can sometimes take up to two years of No Hands training and practice. Only after this awareness has been achieved should practitioners use any of the sharper protuberances of their forearm to achieve deep tissue work. The primary purpose of No Hands Massage is to use this soft front of the forearm to achieve 80% of bodywork. This can and should be done painlessly and effortlessly.

Chapter 25   Benefits

Sources

Everything I claim about No Hands Massage is based on my clinical experiences as a practitioner, a trainer, a supervisor and as a client. Specifically, this means I base the claims I make in this book on what I have learned from:

1   the feedback of my own clients when they report their experiences of No Hands Massage to me and compare these with other bodywork sessions they have received. My clients often make such comparisons spontaneously after their first No Hands session as they are genuinely shocked by the power that this massage form can have on their whole being.

2   my personal comparisons of experiencing bodywork both from those I have trained in No Hands Massage and from bodyworkers untrained in this technique. My comparison of the two has resulted in the realisation that No Hands Massage practitioners of only one or two years experience are proving themselves many times more effective and competent than practitioners with many years conventional bodywork experience behind them.

3   the reported experiences of my many students who have received this style of work from myself and from each other. I regard the reported experiences of one bodyworker who has spent years listening to her body and attempting to articulate those experiences to be worth the feedback of many clients.

4   the feedback that my students' many clients report to them. This new massage system has evolved through training courses and through regular monthly supervision and mentoring groups. This has meant that if anything I teach has not worked, I am still here to receive the feedback. By a process of trial and error, my students and I have identified what works and have discarded or changed that which doesn't work. The groups have been the laboratories in which I have been able to test out my ideas. This book represents the fruits of all our clinical labours and hours and hours of supervisory exploration.

The following are the ten main benefits which I believe result from the diligent learning and practising of No Hands Massage.

1   Increased potency

The full use of the practitioner's body-weight, when combined with the soft front of the forearm and other appropriate parts of the practitioner's body, produces an extremely powerful and deep massage stroke which is experienced as an increase in practitioner potency by the client.

This potent massage can be used equally well with emotionally vulnerable clients who crave gentleness, awareness and sensitivity as it can with sports athletes who sometimes require persistently vigorous, deep and strong work from their practitioners. It is precisely this combination of power and sensitivity which creates an aura of potency around No Hands practitioners. This potency seems also to invite systemic release of tension throughout the client's body, as well as a specific release of the actual muscles or area being worked.

2   Increased protection
- for clients

The strong emphasis placed on the practitioner's own body-movements in No Hands Massage creates a safety in which it is practically impossible for the practitioner to do harm either to themself or the client. When every subtle movement is felt within the practitioner's own body, it is hard to ignore the subtle and less subtle signals from the client's body that something dangerous or damaging is going on. This protection of the client from injury only exists to the extent that the seven postural principles are adhered to. The environment of safety and protection creates a protective atmosphere that is almost palpable and seems to surround the bodywork session.

- for practitioners

At the heart of No Hands Massage is the intention to find ways for bodyworkers to stay bodyworkers into their old age. This can only be achieved if the form of massage not only does no harm to the practitioner, but *actively enhances practitioner health and well being.* Because so many of the new strokes and associated movements have a self-healing and meditative quality to them, as practitioner's we can use this form of massage to actually support our own self healing and enhance our health. Such self healing movements are often slow and considered; another reason why they are experienced by the client as being connected and safe. This increased safety and protection invites a deeper letting go of tension than happens through conventional massage.

3   Healthy practitioner modelling

Protection against harm, when combined with the powerful nature of the movements employed, will ensure that the client experiences bodywork as both effective and safe. The experience of receiving bodywork from a practitioner who clearly displays such physical awareness and attunement will also encourage the client to release their own physical tensions and holding patterns in whatever way they need - be it physically, emotionally, energetically or even spiritually. This is a powerful message to communicate to the client through our touch and our movements. As we move with care and awareness, we model to our clients that letting go is safe.

I believe this principle of modelling can be observed when watching the spirited and lively movements of an audience emerging from a ballet in which they have witnessed movements of grace, beauty and freedom. I believe all bodyworkers need to become dancers in order to model freedom and awareness of movement to their clients.

> *I once demonstrated No Hands Massage on stage to an audience of approximately 200 people at a Mind Body & Spirit conference. At the end, I asked those members of the audience who felt any freer or lighter in their bodies after observing 15 minutes of this form to raise their hands. Over 90% did so.*

Another advantage is that such modelling means that the client will not tolerate any inferior or damaging bodywork in the future. No Hands Massage provides the client with a 'cellular lesson' in looking after and nurturing themself. Once such a powerful form of bodywork is experienced, it is never forgotten. This means that wherever No Hands Massage is available, practitioners of the technique are under pressure to raise their standards and protect themselves from injury. I see this as a good thing for the profession.

4   **Increased permission**

When a bodyworker moves and breathes creatively and freely from their own Hara, they communicate in numerous subliminal ways that it is OK to live and breathe freely and joyfully in their body. This is a profound *permission* that we give to our clients, and a valuable modelling. The permission can then be utilised by the client to fend off the years of childhood training they may have received in muscular and kinaesthetic restriction and tension, namely their inhibiting 'body-script'.

5   **Whole body use - the 'Tao' of No Hands**

The practitioner learns to dance through each massage in a way which is attuned both to themselves and to the client. This Tai Chi dance means that we never get stuck in rigid postures. The bodywork flows in an elemental fashion which is in harmony with the elemental movements of Earth, Air, Fire and Water within each body. This not only makes the bodywork a more powerful healing experience for the client, but ensures the practitioner's own self-healing as well.

Gone are the days of pointless, damaging and often patronising self-sacrifice. Such Victorian principles of 'caring' are replaced with more profoundly spiritual concepts of giving in which the 'giver' and the 'receiver' become indistinguishable. What we see instead, is a slow, grounded and centred movement which enables practitioner and client alike to share in the healing 'now' of each moment - I call this the 'Tao' of No Hands.

6   **Increased endurance (daily)**

If we employ the principles outlined in this book, bodywork becomes an easy and pleasurable experience, rather like enjoying a gentle aerobic work out at a gym, a yoga stretching class and a Tai Chi meditation session all in one. This makes it possible, if we choose, to do more sessions for more days without any exhaustion. Indeed it is possible to postulate that more sessions equals greater self healing. For myself, giving a massage session is often the only time of stillness and healing time that I have amongst all the demands of a young family and a busy schedule.

The absence of excess effort during each massage session, makes each massage a rejuvenating experience for the practitioner. It is not just a case of reducing the amount of tiredness, it is a complete reversal of the psychology of "having to suffer for one's art". This is why so many practitioners of No Hands Massage at my centre can be seen going into their first massage of the day looking tired and heavy in their movements, and can then be observed bouncing around full of life after the session and for the rest of the day!

This is a system which challenges many beliefs common to those of us working in the caring professions. The truth is that by following the postural disciplines outlined earlier, the healing will look after itself. I am a firm believer that it is not the personality of the bodyworker or the amount of effort put into the 'caring' which creates the benefits of bodywork and touch. Instead, I believe it is the excellent practice of *form* that imparts all the benefits of bodywork to our clients.

7   The focus on 'form'

As a bodyworker, my one task is to concentrate on the excellent practice of my *form*. This leaves any healing or therapy to the intrinsic power within the form itself, not to me. It removes my ego from the therapy and allows plenty of space for the client to interact with this form in the most healing way possible for them at this moment in time. I believe that this attention to the actual practice of a bodywork *form* acts as a boundary or a filter which protects both client and practitioner from any over involvement at the psychological level. If I practise this bodywork form well, the healing or the therapy of the client will take care of itself. This is why No Hands practitioners are not tired after sessions, but rejuvenated.

Paradoxically, whilst the practice of No Hands Massage means the practitioner can massage deeply for a much longer time, and could easily extend the session beyond an hour, clients actually experience the session as complete after as little as 30 minutes. I believe that this is because of the power of the deep and gentle strokes.

In addition, more of the client's body is worked with each stroke than in conventional massage. The sheer weight of pressure produces deeper work and the larger surface area of the practitioner's forearms creates massive sensory stimulation. For this reason, I believe that five minutes of No Hands Massage is equivalent to 10 minutes of conventional massage.

The psychological and energetic profundity of this work also means the client does not notice the transit of time. Clients often express surprise at the disparity between their own sense of having had a slow unhurried session which was deep and thorough, and the clock telling them that in fact only 30 minutes has passed. This has enormous implications for practitioners working in half hour slots and in pressured environments.

8 Increased endurance (years)

Through the prevention of wrist damage and the self-healing effects mentioned earlier, we are able to reduce the daily wear and tear on our own bodies. In fact, we are reversing the process into a cycle of rejuvenation. I intend to be a healthier and more effective bodyworker when an octogenarian than I am now. Apart from the joy and pleasure my work creates for me and my clients, the disciplined practice of No Hands Massage represents a sensible investment of my time and energy.

Any hand tension I have accumulated from over-use is eased away by letting each client massage my strained forearm with their body! The muscles that tense up through excessive and unnecessary use of the hands are the very same forearm muscles which get massaged when we employ the techniques introduced in this book. This ensures a long and healthy practice.

All practitioners know that the best marketing tool available is the quality of their work being publicised by word of mouth. The longer I am able to massage, the better I get. The longer I am around, the more chance there is for my clients to talk about me, and for potential new clients to hear about my work.

9 Open heart connection

When seeing many clients for many years it is possible to lose compassion for the people who have come to us for help. Yet compassion is the most powerful therapeutic technique going. It is certainly still the greatest bodywork technique that I know.

It is always valuable to look for ways to keep our hearts open to both ourselves and to our clients. In my opinion, it is not excessive compassion which causes burn out, but rather a closing down of our compassion for ourselves and others. The special movements of No Hands Massage provide us with opportunities to connect with and increase our innate human compassion. This is because most of the forearm techniques used involve a physical exercising and opening of the practitioners own chest area - the zone of the heart Chakra. Many of the movements are similar to Tai-Chi and Chi Kung exercises for opening the heart Chakra and the chest region.

10   Greater intimacy

We all need and seek intimacy. It is a fundamental human need. Most of the new strokes detailed in this book bring the practitioner into much closer physical proximity to the client than does conventional bodywork. Even osteopaths, when wrapping themselves around the client during manipulations only do so for a few seconds. The No Hands practitioner on the other hand is in close proximity to the client *for the whole session*. This can create a more profound client-practitioner bond.

Through my trust of the client (to support my weight), and through the client's trust of me (to let me lean on them), a greater rapport and a closer therapeutic bond is built. Studies have shown that it is precisely this client-practitioner relationship that has been found to be what *clients themselves attribute* to the reasons for their 'cure'.

No Hands Massage, then, is the therapy *par excellence* of intimacy. Bodyworkers speak and talk the language of intimacy through touch. If massage professionals are to lay claim to expertise in any particular area, this is it.

This intimacy of No Hands Massage brings with it a greater need to understand and to keep firm the professional boundaries between ourselves and our clients. It becomes even more important to keep these boundaries clear and to use clear contracts to define our relationship. With such a clear definition of our relationship, the intimacy and strength of bond makes it possible for our clients to effortlessly unravel the sources of their dis-ease through bodywork.

NOTES

Notes on Chapter 1
From Technique to Therapy

1   Information regarding the history of massage was drawn from the following sources:

Benjamin, P *Massage Therapy in the 1940's and the College of Swedish Massage in Chicago, Mass.*, Therapy Journal, 1993

Taylor G H *A sketch of the movement cure 1860* - reprinted in Massage Therapy Journal, 1993

Tracey C *Massage, then and now* Massage Journal 7(3) 10-12, 1992/3

Van der Why, R P *Charles Fayette Taylor* Massage Therapy Journal 32, 1994

Van der Why, R P *History of Massage and its relevance to today's practitioner, the Bodywork Knowledgebase*, self published, New York, 1992

2   The list of massage authors who have contributed to the understanding of massage is enormous, and would include, among others:

Bohm, M *Massage: its principles and technique* Saunders, 1913

Cassar, M *Handbook of Massage Therapy* Butterworth Heineman, 1999

Cyriax, E J *Deep Massage and Manipulation Illustrated* Hamish Hamilton Med Books, 1947

Dicke, E *Meine Bindegewebmassage* Hippocrates-Verlag, 1956

Fritz, S *Fundamentals of Therapeutic Massage* Mosby, 2000 (2nd Ed)

Greenman, P E *Principles of Manual Medicine* Williams and Wilkin, 1989

Juhan, D *Job's Body - a handbook for Bodywork* Station Hill Press, 1987

Kellog, J H *The Art of Massage* Battle Creek, Mich Modern Medicine Publishing, 1929

McMillan, M. *Massage and Therapeutic Exercises* Saunders, 1932 (3rd Ed)

Mennell James, M A *Massage, its principles and practise*, 1920

Tappan, F *Healing Massage Techniques. Holistic, Classic and Emerging Methods* Appleton & Lange, 1988 (2nd Ed)

Tappan, F *Massage Techniques - a case method approach* Macmillan, New York, 1961

Yates, J *Physiological Effects of Therapeutic Massage* Therapists Association of British Columbia, 1989

3   There are many advanced and new approaches to western bodywork, most of which
      rely on the hands as their primary tool of treatment. A brief list that is not
      exhaustive would include the following publications:
      Chaitow L *Soft Tissue Manipulation* Thorsons, 1987
      Ebner, M *Connective Tissue Massage* Drieger, New York, 1962
      Ingham, E *The Ingham Reflex Method of Compression Massage* Ingham Publications,
      1959
      Pfrimmer, T *Muscles - your invisible bonds* Vantage, New York, 1970
      Rolf, I P *Rolfing, the integration of the human structure* Harper & Row, 1977
      Stone, R *Polarity Therapy, the complete collected works* Reno, NV:CRCS Publications,
      1986
      Travell, J G & Simmons, D G *Myofascial Pain and Dysfunction* Williams &
      Wilkins, 1983 (trigger point therapy)
      Wittlinger, G & Wittlinger, H. *Dr Vodder's Manual Lymph Drainage* Heidelberg
      Karl Haug, 1970

4   There are so many who have contributed to the diversity and creativity of bodywork
      over the last century that it becomes impossible to list them all in a short space. See
      my article *Massage History*, Shi'Zen Publications, 2000 for a tentative list.

5   The value of touch and its mental and emotional effect can be reviewed through the
      following:
      Lowen, A *Bioenergetics* Penguin, 1976
      Millenson, J *Mind Matters, psychological medicine in holistic practise* Seattle Eastland
      Press, 1995
      Montagu, A *Touching, the human significance of the skin* Harper & Row, 1986 (3rd
      Ed)
      Older, J *Touching is Healing* Stein & Day, New York, 1982
      Reich, W *The Function of the Orgasm* London, 1968
      Selye, H *The Stress of Life* McGraw Hill, 1984
      Tisserand, R *Success with Stress* International Journal of Aromatherapy, 1992
      Summer

6   An excellent summary of the profession's struggle to become regulated can be found
      in Fritz, S *Fundamentals of Therapeutic Massage* Mosby, 2000 (2nd Ed), (p.16-23).
      Such regulation is still a hot debate in the pages of massage magazines in the USA.

Notes On Chapter 2
Squaring the Circle - The Postural Problems of Bodywork

1   Beck (1988, p.388), Thomas (1987, p.19,) and Cassar (1999, p.15) particularly
     highlight the need for oriental approaches to stance and movement in order to
     reduce injury. Fritz (1995, p.177-190) uses these same approaches, though she
     describes them in much more scientific and western language.

2   Such approaches have their origins in the stances and movements of oriental martial
     arts, where a good posture was quite literally a matter of life and death Reid (1994)
     and Chuen (1991). The west has also made significant contributions towards
     posture, that are relevant to today's practitioner. These can be found in the
     literature and trainings established through the work of Frederick Alexander (1955)
     and Moshe Feldenkrais (1980).

3   Regarding what constitutes a 'full practise', Beck (1988, p.335) states that: *"A
     professional massage therapist will perform six to ten treatments each day.".* Fritz (1995,
     p.177) concurs by stating that a practitioner should be able to do eight hours
     massage a day, and she goes on to say: *"To make a full time living doing bodywork,
     the practitioner must be able to give 15 to 30 sessions per week.".* Cash (1996) states
     that *"a busy therapist may do perhaps eight or more treatments a day"* and that *"a
     treatment may take an hour".*

4   There are many examples of this approach to reducing practitioner damage:
     Cassar (1999, p. 31, fig 2.27), Fritz (1995, p.250, fig 10.16c and p.239, fig 10.7),
     Cash (1996, p.180), Beck (1988, p.309, fig 10.3), Holey and Cook (1997, p.162)

5   Many examples of bodywork which are stressful to the wrists, thumb and fingers of
     the practitioner may be found in even a cursory glance through any bodywork
     book. Specific examples can be seen in: Cassar (p.23, fig 2.15), Cash (p.134), Beck
     (p.426) and Fritz (p.247, fig 10.14).

6   Fritz (1995, p.184) states that *"grasping manipulations, such as petrissage are stressful
     on the hands.".*

7   Again, many examples of this can be found in any bodywork book. Specific examples include: Cassar (1999, p.103, fig 5.17), Fritz (1995, p.192, fig 8.19), Cash (1996, p.193), Beck (1988, p.309, fig 10.3).

8   Fritz (1995, p.181, fig 8.4) in showing good posture of the practitioner's body and in bothering to discuss the vectors of force at play during a massage stroke, demonstrates visually the forces imposed on the wrist joint.

9   Cassar (1999, p.97, and p.98, fig 5.1) demonstrates extensive clinical use of what he calls 'Du Pong' techniques or 'knuckling'. Examples of this fist technique can also be seen in Fritz (1995, p.228, fig 10.1).

Notes on Chapter 3
Bodywork and Injury

1   The adjusted equation, $Z = NH + AF + T = E$ is a mnemonic tool aimed at highlighting the difference one small change can make. It is a simplification that focuses on the winning formula for practitioner body-use. Effective bodywork, of course, requires much more than postural efficiency and zero damage to the practitioner. It also requires clinical experience, knowledge, clear contracting, sensitivity and intuition, all of which zero-strain bodywork will help produce.

Notes on Chapter 4
Assessing Your Practice

1   As far as I am aware, such timed stroke analysis is an original concept in massage assessment and could be usefully employed in massage schools to create awareness of body-use.

2   The Tibetan Chakra system already shows the centre of the palms of the hands as containing an important energy or Chakra centre. Many teachers and authors on energy and healing draw attention to this unique aspect of the hands. Chuen (1991)

Notes on Chapter 9
Postural Principle Flow

1   Regarding the effect that images held in our minds can have on the way we move, a great deal of sport psychology centres around the use of visualisation to alter performance.

Kent (1994) identifies the use of 'imagery' and 'external imagery' in the acquisition of skills. David Hemery surveyed 50 world class performers and found creativity, visualisation and imagery to be at the core of their excellence, and that *"they all regarded such visualisations to have contributed to the successful execution of their sport".* Hemery (1991).

Silva III & Weinberg in 'Psychological Foundations of Sport' state that: *"There seems to be little doubt that mental practise can positively affect skilled motor performance...."* and use the term 'kinesthetic imagery' (p.153) to describe visualisations which involve sensory experiences of the performer.

Bull, S J in his 'Sport Psychology' states that *"visualisation works because it helps establish the correct blueprint for success"* (p.88).

Within the realms of psychotherapy, such visualisation work was pioneered by Erickson (1967) and developed by many later writers. Utilising positive images is one of the hallmarks of Neuro-Linguistic Programming, a modern synthesis of much that was found to be effective in psychotherapy Bandler & Grinder (1979). More specifically in the bodywork field, Feldenkrais (1980) advocated the use of images to achieve balanced poise and self-healing.

In the field of dance, a striking example of the use of images based on pure energy can be found in the choreography of Merce Cunningham. His revolutionary new dance form was not unsurprisingly accompanied by a new and flowing approach to choreographic notation. Rather than use the more conventional static images of his day, he used dynamic and flowing imagery. His imagery conveys the spirit and essence of the movements as much as the form, and resembles oriental paintings more than any western art forms. 'The Dancer and the Dance' Merce Cunningham in conversation with Jacqueline Lesschaeve (p.14-15)

2   Regarding the literature on the principle and effectiveness of Flow, many authors make reference to the importance of this concept:

Cassar states that: *"When all the scientific theory on massage movements has been studied and absorbed, what remains is the art of the techniques."* He regards this 'art' as being related to rhythm, and that this rhythm *"increases stroke effectiveness"*. He goes on to say: *"It is also important to mention that establishing a good rhythm to the overall treatment helps the practitioner to focus and tune into the recipient, which underlines that the treatment is more about healing the patient than the tissues".*

Clearly writing from his own clinical experience, he then identifies that such rhythm (or flow) can have a powerful impact on the depth of bodywork given: *"Furthermore, when the therapist is relaxed and working to a rhythm the treatment can be expanded to include other aspects – ie the energy and subconscious levels.".* *Handbook of Massage Therapy (1999 p.18).*

Regarding the dangers of injury if flow is not attained by the practitioner, Cassar states that: *"comfort and ease of movement are very significant if mechanical stress on the body is to be avoided".* *Handbook of Massage Therapy (1999 p.13).*

Beck hints at this energetic dimension to posture and its impact on both the client and the practitioner, when he states that good 'whole body' posture helps sustain energy and *"enables the practitioner to move around the table more freely and easily while maintaining the flow of movement and energy".* He also shows awareness that the antithesis of flow can be dangerous to the practitioner by pointing out that *"stiff rigid knees contribute to fatigue, while locking the knees forces a posture that puts the back in danger of injury".* *Theory and Practise of Therapeutic Massage (1988, p.336, p. 338).*

Cash identifies the potency which can result from effective posture when he states that with a *"good working posture. . . massage becomes effortless, instinctive and extremely powerful".* *Sport and Remedial Massage Therapy, (1996, p.29).*

Fritz 1995 shows a clinician's instinctive awareness of this dance-like movement when she says *"If the proper body mechanics are used, the therapist will look and feel relaxed and graceful while giving a massage.".* *Fundamentals of Therapeutic Massage (1995, p.179).*

3   Regarding the significance that the practitioner's movement can have on clients, Smith-Artaud in *'Dance Composition'*, states that: *"It should be clear that movement is a vast communication language and that varieties of combinations of its elements constitute many thousands of movement 'words'."*. (p.17)

Whilst Smith-Artaud is writing about dancers, the same is true of massage practitioners, who 'talk' to their clients in the basic language of movement.

Cheney, in '*Basic Concepts in Modern Dance*' identifies that *"most of your basic knowledge came to you through movement. . . You first experienced yourself by the movement of your body."* (p.14).

The power of movement to communicate probably reached its most famous in the stunningly moving and creative dances of Nureyev. '*Nureyev - his spectacular early years. An autobiography*'.

4   Many books on oriental medicine, Tai Chi and other martial arts refer to the inner strength that can be gathered through disciplined, flowing movements. They also refer to the interplay between the sensitivity and awareness of the practitioner and the healing power that can result.

Cheun writes of Chi Kung "What began as a search for health becomes a process of self-healing. Having learned how to heal ourselves, we are then able to help others" (1999, p.110) '*The Way of Healing.*'

and that *"The more you have been able to release the blocked chi within you. . . the more effective you will be in healing yourself and others."* (1991, p.188) '*The Way of Energy*'

Masunaga (1977, p.6, p.7) states that: *"In both Zen and shiatsu we are dealing with something that cannot be explained rationally but that should be felt by the living body. . . In shiatsu simply pressing will not reveal to you the life essence of what you are pressing. . . By applying your hand on a point or tsubo and following the Meridian lines with your fingers, you may feel the "echo" of life. If you can receive and understand this sensation, disease will seem to disappear."* '*Zen Shiatsu*'

Lauriann Greene (1995) states that: *"the massage practitioner must see herself as a massage athlete."*.

In bodywork literature, Cash considers the athletic role of a bodyworker when he states *"massage is a very physical therapy and as such can almost be considered a sport in itself"* *'Sport and Remedial Massage Therapy'* (1996, p.26)

5   Regarding the practitioner sensing subtle movements of energy within the client's body, the principles of Cranio Sacral Therapy are based on the practitioner being able to feel these. Upledger, J E and Vredevoogd, J *'Craniosacral Therapy'* Seattle, Eastland Press (1983)

NOTES on Chapter 11
Postural Principle Five   Supported Massage

1   Many bodywork writers (Cassar, Beck etc) have identified this surprisingly powerful oriental stance as important for the practitioner's own postural training and awareness. When combined with exercises which encourage movement with one or both knees bent, we produce bodywork movements of awareness, power, and sensitivity. Beck (p.338), Cassar

Notes on Chapter 12
Postural Principle Six   Kneeling

1   The notion of massaging upwards was, unsurprisingly, first put into print by Fritz, one of the most significant contributors to a clear description of therapeutic massage posture. She describes this from either a standing technique which she calls "leaning uphill" (p.263. 2000), or a sitting position (p.260). In neither case are the strokes performed with a vertical back - this was not her focus. Where I differ from Fritz, is in the lowering of the massage table and applying upward strokes from kneeling, without leaning, with the stroke being powered by the hips keeping a vertical back.

Notes on Chapter 15
The Philosophy of No Hands Massage

1 Don McFarland *'Body Secrets'* states *"My present understanding of pain is that it is totally counterproductive. The only time I give pain now is when I don't know enough **not** to give pain, or when I neglect to listen to the body before me. I consider pain to be my fault completely, never my client's.*

Even if my client is resistive to change, if I can listen closely enough to his body I can slip past the resistances."

Notes on Chapter 16
Seven Psychological Principles

1 In Transactional Analysis, a "one up" position is when I regard myself as more superior and important than my client, where I am 'OK' and the client is 'Not OK'. A "one down" position is where I regard my client as superior and more important than me, where I am 'Not OK' and the client is 'OK'. Berne (1966)

BIBLIOGRAPHY

Alternative Medicine: Expanding Medical Horizons: A report to the National Institutes on Health on Alternative medical Systems and Practices in the United States, 1994

Adams, A *Degenerative Masseurs Syndrome* workshop presentation, 2000

Alexander F *The Use of the Self* London Re-educational Publications, 1955

Anderson, J *Art Without Boundaries* Dance Books Ltd, 1997

Bandler, R and Grinder, J *Frogs Into Princes* Real People Press, 1979

Beck, M F *Milady's Theory and Practise of Therapeutic Massage* Milady Publishing Company, 1988 (2nd Ed)

Berne, E *Games People Play* Deutsch Books, 1966

Bull, S J *Sport Psychology, a self-help guide* The Crowood Press Ltd, 1991

Calhoun, D W *Sport, Culture and Personality* Human Kinetics Publishers Inc, 1987

Casement, P *On Learning from the Patient* London, Tavistock, 1985

Cash, M *Sports and Remedial Massage Therapy,* Ebury Press, 1996

Cassar, M-P *Handbook of Massage Therapy,* Butterworth-Heinemann, 1999

Cassar, M-P *Massage Made Easy* Quarto Publishing plc, 1996

Cheney, G *Basic Concepts in Modern Dance, a creative approach* Princeton Book Company, 1989 (3rd Ed)

Chuen, L K *The Way of Energy* Gaia Books, 1991

Cunningham, M *The Dancer and the Dance*   Marion Boyars Inc, 1985

Davies, D *Psychological Factors in Competitive Sport* The Falmer Press, 1989

Dorland, S Pocket Medical Dictionary W B Saunders Company Ltd, 1982

Ericson, M H *The Collected Papers. . . on Hypnosis*, New York, Irvington (1980)

Eyerman, K *Massage* Sidgwick & Jackson, London, 1987

Feldenkrais, M *Awareness Through Movement, health exercises for personal growth* Penguin Arkana, 1980

Fritz, S *Mosby's Fundamentals of Therapeutic Massage* Mosby Lifeline 1995

Fritz, S *Mosby's Fundamentals of Therapeutic Massage* Mosby Inc 2000 (2nd Ed)

Greene, L *Save Your Hands* self published, 1995

Hemery, D *Sporting Excellence, what makes a champion?* Collins Willow (HarperCollins), 1991

Holey and Cook *Therapeutic Massage* W B Saunders Company Ltd, 1997

Kent, M *The Oxford Dictionary of Sports Science and Medicine* Oxford University Press, 1994

Lundberg, P *The Book of Shiatsu, vitality and health through the art of touch* Gaia Books Ltd, 1992

Masunaga, S and Wataru, C *Zen Shiatsu, how to harmonize Yin and Yan for better health* Japan Publications Inc, 1977

Masunaga, S *Meridian Exercises* Japan Publications Inc, 1987

Nureyev, R *Nureyev, His Spectacular Early Years* Hodder & Stoughton Ltd, 1962

Porter, R Professor of History of Medicine, Welcome Trust, UK, personal communication, 2000

Pyves, G *Massage History* Shi'Zen Publications, 2000

Reid, H *The Book of Soft Martial Arts* Gaia Books, 1994

Seward, D *Understanding Stuctures* Macmillan, 1998

Silva 111, J M and Weinberg, R S (editors) *Psychological Foundations of Sport* Human Kinetics Books, 1984

Smith-Autard, J M *Dance Composition* A&C Black (Publishers) Ltd, 1996 (3rd Ed)

Solomon, E P *Introduction to Human Anatomy and Physiology* W B Saunders Company Ltd, 1992

Solomon, E P, Schmidt R R and Adragna, P J *Human Anatomy and Physionlogy* Saunders (2nd Ed), 1983

Stone, R J and Stone J A *Atlas of the Skeletal Muscles* Wm C Brown, 1996

Tappan, F M *Healing Massage Techniques, holistic, classic and emerging methods* Appleton & Lange, 1988

Thie, J F *Touch for Health* Devorss & Company, 1989 (revised expanded edition)

Thomas, S *Massage for Common Ailments* Gaia Books, 1989

University of Exeter's Centre for Complementary Health Studies *Professional organisation of complementary and alternative medicine in the United Kingdom* (1997): A report to the department of Health

Vickers, A, Van Toller, S and Stevensen, C *Massage and Aromatherapy, a guide for health professionals* Chapman & Hall, 1996

Woods, B *Applying Psychology to Sport* Hodder & Stoughton Educational, 1998

GLOSSARY OF TERMS

Anatomical directions

Wherever possible I have tried to use non-medical jargon, adding the following terms in parentheses for clarity:

Anterior

The front of the body, in front of, before. For example, the abdomen is on the anterior side: the stomach is anterior to the spine. An illustration or observation showing the front of the body or of a region is referred to as the anterior view. A direction of a massage movement towards the front of the body is said to be in an anterior direction, or anteriorly.

Caudad or caudal

Caudad is from the Latin *cauda*, meaning 'tail', and *ad*, meaning 'towards'; opposite to cephalad. A similar work is caudal, from the Latin *caudalis*, meaning 'pertaining to the tail'. The term refers to the location of a body organ or region which is situated nearer to the 'tail' (coccyx) than a particular reference point - for example, the abdomen is caudad to the chest. This is in some ways synonymous with the term 'inferior'.

Caudad or caudal is also used to indicate a direction which is towards the posterior aspect of the body, and can be used for a movement or to indicate that an organ lies deeper inside the abdomen or below another organ (therefore more posteriorly). The term is employed to describe the direction of a massage movement when it is carried out towards the pelvis or the feet.

Another application is to specify which hand is needed for a particular movement - for example, 'the caudad hand (the one nearest to the patient's feet) applies to effleurage whilst the cephalad hand (the one nearest to the patient's head) stabilises the limb'.

Centrifugal

From the Greek *kentron*, meaning 'centre' and the Latin *fugere*, meaning 'to flee'. Describes a movement moving away from the centre and towards the periphery.

Centripetal

From the Greek *kentron*, meaning 'centre', and the Latin *petere*, meaning to 'seek'. Describes a movement towards the centre of the body from the periphery.

Cephalad or cephalic

From the Greek word *kephale*, meaning 'head'; opposite to caudad. A similar word is cephalic, from the Latin *cephalus*, meaning 'cranial' or 'pertaining to the head'. The term is also synonymous with 'superior', and indicates the position of an organ or region which is closer to the head than a particular reference point - for example, the chest is cephalad to the abdomen. In this text, the term is used to describe the direction of a massage movement when it is carried out towards the head. It is also utilised to demonstrate which hand is needed for a particular manoeuvre - for example, the caudad hand (the one nearest to the patient's feet) applies the effleurage whilst the cephalad hand (the one nearest to the patient's head) stabilises the limb'.

Contralateral

From the Latin *latus*, meaning 'side'. Indicates the location of a region which is on the opposite side of the midline from the point of reference - for instance, the right side of the spine might be affected by a nerve impulse originating in the contralateral (left) side. In massage, the term is used to indicate the opposite side of the body from where the massage therapist stands.

Coronal plane

See frontal plane.

Distal

From the Latin *distare*, meaning 'to be distant'. Indicates the farthest point away from the centre of the body or from the trunk. The term is mostly used to describe the position of the part of the limb which is farther away from the trunk than the point of reference – for example, the wrist is distal to the elbow.

Frontal plane

A plane which divides the body into the anterior and posterior portions, at right angles to the midsagittal plane.

Hypothenar eminence

The prominent fleshy part of the palm, just below the little finger.

Inferior

The location of a body part or organ which is beneath or deeper to the more superficial point of reference – for instance, the ribs are inferior to the pectoralis muscle group. The term is also used to describe the position of an organ, tissue or bony landmark which is further towards the feet that its point of reference – for example, the inferior border of the iliac crest is further towards the feet than the superior border. This bearing primarily applies when the subject is in the standing posture (anatomical position), but it is equally relevant when lying down. In this context it is synonymous with the term caudad.

Ipsilateral

From the Latin *ipse*, meaning 'the same' and *latus*, meaning 'side'. Indicates the same side of the body as the point of reference – for instance, a reflex action like that of the patellar reflex is created by tapping the patellar tendon just below the knee, which causes contraction of the thigh muscles on the ipsilateral side. In massage it is used to describe a movement carried out on the same side of the body as where the therapist stands.

Midsagittal plane

An imaginary line passing through the body, dividing it into symmetrical halves (right and left).

Medial

Towards the central axis of the body – for example, the medial axis of the femur is in the region of the adductor muscles. The term is also utilised when describing a massage movement, and in this case the medial hand is the one which is positioned nearest to the midline or to the spine of the patient.

The 'lateral' hand is the one which is positioned closer to the lateral border of the body. For instance, when a deep effleurage is applied to the back, the medial hand carries out the movement and it is reinforced with the more lateral hand.

Lateral

Towards the outside of the body – for instance, the lateral aspect of the femur is in the region of the iliotibial band. The term is also used when describing a massage movement (see *medial*, above)

Paravertebral

Alongside or near the vertebral column. This term is frequently used to indicate the muscles of the back which are close to the spine.

Passive movements

These are actions or movements of joints which are carried out by the therapist without any assistance from the subject - for example, the hamstring muscles are stretched passively when the subject is lying supine and the lower limb is raised and flexed at the hip joint by the practitioner.

Periphery

The outer part or outer surface of the body. The peripheral tissues are, therefore, those of the skin and subcutaneous fascia and their integrated soft tissue structures.

Posterior

The back area of the body – for instance, the spine is located on the posterior region of the body.

Prone

When the subject is lying face down.

Proximal

Describes the position of that part of a limb which is nearer to the trunk than the point of reference – for example, the elbow is proximal to the wrist.

Somatic
Meaning, the body.

Superior
The position of a body region or organ which is situated above or higher than the point of reference – for example, the scapula is superior to the ribs. The term is also used to describe the position of an organ, tissue or bony landmark which is farther towards the head than its point of reference – for example, the superior border of the iliac crest is farther up than the inferior border. This bearing primarily applies when the subject is in the standing posture (anatomical position) but it is equally relevant when they are lying down. In this context it is synonymous with the term cephalad.

Supine
Opposite to prone; the body is in the lying down position facing upwards.

Systemic
Pertaining to the whole body rather than to one part.

Thenar eminence
From the Greek thenar, meaning 'palm'. This term refers to the fleshy part of the hand at the base of the thumb; where the abductor and flexor muscles of the thumb itself are located.

Thoracic
Pertaining to the upper back or thoracic spine.

Transverse plane
A plane which transverses the body horizontally at any level.

Anatomical position

The stance of the body when standing erect. This means arms hanging to the side, palms facing forward.

Fascia   Refers to the continuous fibrous sheet that envelopes the body beneath the skin. This 'tissue envelope' encloses muscle groups, and even separates muscle layers. It is the subject of much debate in many bodywork modalities.

Front V   This refers to the V created when you bend your elbow joint. The front (anterior) surface is soft and is useful for mangling and supporting heavy limbs.

Hard back   This refers to the posterior muscle of the forearm (wrist, hand and finger extensors).

Hard point   (of elbow)
This refers to the olecranon.

Inter-phalangeal joints
The joints of the fingers

Posterior V   This refers to the V made between your upper and lower outer arm when you strike your chest. This is useful for transmitting body-weight on to the client.

Small hooks
This refers to the two small bony outcrops at each side of your forearm just below your wrist (the styloid processes of the distal radius and ulna).

Soft front   This refers to the 2- 4 inches of soft, fatty tissue at the "elbow end" of the front of your forearm (the proximal anterior portion of your lower arm). This is the preferred tool for most No Hands Massage. If you use the "wrist end" of your front forearm your movements become more 'bony' and painful to the client. It is also possible, when doing lots of massage with this part of your body, to cause irritation and damage to all the nerves and veins which run superficially at this more vulnerable end of your forearm. (Also referred to as **soft pads**.)

Soft hook   This refers to the medial epicondyle of the humerus.

Soft pads   see Soft front.

Ulnar edge   This refers to the medial shaft of the ulna.

Up leg/ down leg

This refers to the practitioner in a half kneeling position (the proposal stance). In this posture, one knee is 'up' and one is 'down'. These become the 'up' and 'down' legs respectively.

Working hand/arm

This means the hand or arm which is actually applying the movement to the client's body - as distinguished from the other hand, the "non–working" hand or arm. It is meant as a description of the client's experience. In reality the non-working hand/arm may be doing a more important job than the working one. This is most clearly seen when the practitioner is using the non-working hand to "listen" for the client's subtle responses to bodywork.